Neither Married nor Single

WHEN YOUR PARTNER HAS ALZHEIMER'S OR OTHER DEMENTIA

David Kirkpatrick, MA, MD

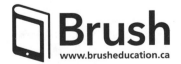

Brush
www.brusheducation.ca

Brush Education Inc.
www.brusheducation.ca
contact@brusheducation.ca
Copy editing: Leslie Vermeer
Cover and interior design: Carol Dragich, Dragich Design; Cover image: istock: stevecoleimages

Excerpts from "Re-Inventing a Life" by Michael Smith reproduced by permission of the author. Page 132: David and Clair, 2008; photographed by joy Fai.

Library and Archives Canada Cataloguing in Publication
Kirkpatrick, David, 1939-, author
        Neither married nor single: when your partner has Alzheimer's or other dementia / Dr. David Kirkpatrick.
Includes bibliographical references.
Issued in print and electronic formats.
ISBN 978-1-55059-728-8 (softcover).--ISBN 978-1-55059-729-5 (PDF).--ISBN 978-1-55059-730-1 (Kindle).--ISBN 978-1-55059-731-8 (EPUB)
        1. Kirkpatrick, David, 1939- --Marriage. 2. Alzheimer's disease--Patients--Care. 3. Alzheimer's disease--Patients--Family relationships. 4. Caregivers. I. Title.

RC523.2.F58 2018   362.1968'31   C2017-906795-8
                                                                        C2017-906796-6

We acknowledge the support of the Government of Canada
Nous reconnaissons l'appui du gouvernement du Canada | Canada

To Clair Ladner Hawes.
You made a difference.

Contents

Preface   ix

Acknowledgements   xi

1   The Diagnosis   1

2   Alzheimer's Disease: A History and an Update   17

3   Finding Help and Comfort for Your AD Partner   33

4   Care Homes   41

5   Improving Your AD Partner's Quality of Life   53

6   Taking Care of the Caregiver   61

7   Sexuality and Intimacy   79

8   Into the Future   109

    Notes   127

    Bibliography   129

    About the Author   132

Preface

There was a time when I laboured under the misconception that Alzheimer's disease and other dementias were tragedies that happened to other people, older people. After all, as a psychologist, a psychiatrist with three years' experience in geriatric psychiatry and—most central to my professional identity—a psychotherapist for more than thirty years, I had been counselling the victims of dementia in its many guises, as well as the caregivers whose lives had been completely disrupted by it.

Then in 2007 my wife, Clair, a gifted clinical psychologist, was diagnosed with early-onset Alzheimer's disease. As her life changed and deteriorated, my life changed, too. But I found myself experiencing her tragedy as a sort of outsider-insider. On the one hand I was a curious, detached clinician; on the other, I was a heartbroken, grieving partner looking for help like any other caregiver of a partner struggling with this intruder.

I soon learned that almost all the literature on Alzheimer's is written for people caring for parents or grandparents with the disease, not for partners and caregivers within an Alzheimer's marriage. Yes, there are great books of fiction and movies exploring the married perspective, but I was looking for a true story told from both a personal and a professional point of view. As Clair's disease progressed, I documented her story in my daily journals. One day I began to write that story down formally—for myself, at first, and then for a wider audience as I realized how many other women and men in Alzheimer's marriages were seeking help.

From about 2010 to 2014 I belonged to a support group for Alzheimer's and other dementias. Several friends from this group, along with a few others, responded warmly to my request for discussions and informal recall of their experiences with their loved ones with dementia. We talked, listened and shared in confidence, so their real names do not appear in this book.

With this encouragement, I began exploring and writing about some of the topics that caregiving partners—and even dementia support groups!—generally tiptoe around in order to avoid offending families and friends: When is the right time to find or even begin considering a care home for your loved one? What is a "normal" sex life with an Alzheimer's partner? When is it appropriate to consider re-socializing with a new partner? Can I/may I love two people at once without incurring the righteous anger, resentment or frustration of friends or family—or, heaven forbid, both?

And so my manuscript gradually evolved into a "how-to" for the caregiving partners of dementia sufferers, a book that offers a hand to those of you who live within an Alzheimer's (or other dementia) partnership. It is not written to make you feel happier or to cheer you up, but to help you nurture, develop and experience the real you. And as you read on, I hope you will find yourself moving far beyond the emptiness of grief that dementia has brought into your life.

You are not alone.

Acknowledgements

Thank you

To Betty Keller and Leslie Vermeer, whose combined sense of editorial clarity stopped short of sentimentality and made this book the best it could possibly be.

To my gifted home office manager, joy Fai, who truly made a difference before and after Clair's diagnosis and kept our respective offices humming without fail.

To my children and step-children, Andy, Christy, Mindy and Stefan, who supported Clair, me and both of us without ever complaining.

To therapists Molly and Grant. To Dr. Jeff Beckman.

To friends and family, Jay and Florina. Sara and Shmuel. Susan and Maggie. Stephy and Dan. And Edie, Susan and Doug.

To all the staff at Kiwanis Care Centre, who looked after Clair for six years with devotion, warmth and professionalism.

And to Clair's patients and clients, who never forgot her but remember her with sharp gratitude and appreciation.

To the members of our dementia support groups and those who volunteered their time to talk with me of their experiences.

To the millions of individuals in this world struggling with Alzheimer's and other forms of dementia today.

And to their family, friends, caregivers and communities who continue their nurturance of these individuals with love, courage, commitment and persistence.

CHAPTER ONE

The Diagnosis

It was March 2007 and my wife Clair and I had endured what seemed like an excruciating, unnecessarily long period of diagnostic frustration, awaiting some answers—any answers—to what was plaguing her. Brief lapses in memory. Losing her keys—but shoot, I'd done that myself more than once. Misinterpreting others' actions and reactions. Mild disorganization such as leaving bedroom and bathroom lights on—I did that, too—and trying to bake a pizza in the microwave. But all of this was way out of character for the highly organized woman I had known and loved for more than twelve years.

Now the results of her visit to the neuropsychologist had been relayed to her neurologist, and we sat waiting for him to pass on the news.

"It's TIAs, isn't it?" the anxious physician within me asked hopefully. TIA stands for *transient ischemic attack*, which is a small, often temporary stroke.

The neurologist shook his head slowly but surely. Then he quietly explained that my wife had Alzheimer's disease or, as he diplomatically shortened it, *AD*. Before we left his office, he wrote her a prescription for memantine, one of the four or five medications that help slow, though not stop, the progress of this relentlessly cruel and pitiless memory-killer. As we drove back to our home on Vancouver's north shore, my wife began crying quietly.

"Do you want to share?" I asked at a stoplight.

"Well, you've been through this before," she observed, referring to the cancer death of my wife Betsy.

"Well, you have too, honey," I said, a reminder that she had lost her first husband to pancreatic cancer. We were mostly quiet as we drove the rest of the way home, our private, probably overlapping thoughts, fears and fantasies swirling in our respective heads.

|||||||||||||||||||||||||||||||||

Clair was suffering from early-onset Alzheimer's disease. It had first been symptomatic five years earlier, when she was only sixty-two, an age at which very few in the general population are so unfairly stricken. A gifted clinical psychologist, she had been in steady demand in those days to give workshops to counsellors and psychologists working in the field, professionals who wanted to take further instruction from someone with such an outstanding and deserved international reputation. But there had been little incidents that indicated all was not right with her: missed appointments, confusion over a passport renewal, misinterpretations of family and colleagues' actions. On February 21, 2002, she had written in her journal:

> So much is happening that I can't keep issues straight . . . Every one of these hiccups seems to take the stuffing out of me. And I am so tired . . . We took [grandson] William for the weekend . . . He kept us busy & David seemed annoyed/irritated that he was there . . . I was picking up black vibes from David [which] was not helping because amongst other things, as he saw it, no sex. But he was creating an unpleasant aura . . . Everything seems to be compounded by my forgetfulness—e.g., I asked Mary to pick up the signed passport application [at J's clinic], and she did so— at least she went there but I had not yet taken it [there] . . . I try to stay/be organized but I have never felt so disorganized. Passport papers, insurance papers. This leads to much pain. Worrying if dementia is setting in. I need more time.

After presenting a week-long workshop in London in July 2004, Clair emailed me, adding a very pleased note that her hostess "was thrilled with the card holder, in pewter and pearl, that I gave her . . . Actually, I forgot to give it to her [when I arrived] and found it in my suitcase when I packed this morning." It was an innocent postscript, but it was a reminder that in a somewhat synchronous fashion we had both been pushing our respective fears and anxieties about her health into the background and continuing to love, appreciate and fully enjoy each other.

Then in late spring 2006 Clair returned to the United Kingdom to teach, and what happened during that trip would tell each of us that ours was going to be a more challenging marriage than either of us had imagined. In a message I received on June 4, she explained that she had told her friend and host about her health issues. "Because [she] was originally a speech therapist, she knew quite a bit about brain functioning. So we had a good chat. I am now very tired." The next day she emailed me.

> It seems like forever since I saw you, made love with you, felt so safe with you. It was good that I had told [her hostess] about the problems I have been having . . . [because] this morning I have had total mind/memory blanks . . . It makes me feel sad to be so out of touch with myself . . . I am hoping this all has to do with jet lag. Please be assured that I am in good hands and that my friends are so very supportive. I plan to go for a walk this afternoon and maybe clear my head.

On June 15 I received a phone call from Clair's concerned hostess and colleague to say that Clair's mind/memory blanks had increased. Afterwards I spoke with Clair, then emailed back to her hostess:

> Talked with Clair at about 0845 your time. She was understandably upset, reminded me her [reviews from workshop participants in Wales] were uniformly okay, all "5/5 except for two 4/5s!" but she did try to listen to my concerns. I think she will . . . cancel balance of her trip but am not sure. Faxing her MDs today.

Three days later I heard back from Clair's hostess:

> Dear David,
>
> I would really appreciate the opportunity to talk to you about how Clair is doing and my concerns about her going to Greece and then later to Green Park. Could you get back to me as soon as possible with your number and when I could best catch you? It has been wonderful to spend time with Clair and we have had a great time together in Cambridge and in Wales. However, her difficulties are very marked—more than I think she is aware, although I know she is understandably very anxious and distressed about her challenges with short term memory and spatial/time awareness.
>
> Hope to talk with you very soon.

Clair's trip to Greece was cancelled, and her teaching tour of Europe was cut short. She returned home to Canada frustrated. Like me, she was puzzled and anxious about this turn of events in her life, but she was also cooperative, eager to help us help her. We assured ourselves that things must be getting better, right? That we would discuss the problem tomorrow—or when it was quiet. Each of us in our own way was eager for answers, wanting to make sense of these pieces to our shared puzzle. Then in the spring of 2007 we received the answer we were dreading: Alzheimer's disease.

A week or so after we received the verdict from the neurologist, Clair insisted we see the movie *Away from Her*, which had been adapted from an Alice Munro short story called "The Bear Came over the Mountain." The film covers a time of transition in the lives of an Alzheimer's-afflicted woman (played by Julie Christie) and her retired college professor husband (played by Gordon Pinsent) as they struggle together and separately with the themes of socialization, relationship possibilities and needs, sexuality, commitment, intimacy, loneliness and loyalty. The husband experiences an epiphany when the wife transfers her affections to another man, a wheelchair-bound mute who is a patient in the same care home. Clair and I laughed. We cried. Afterward we shared our feelings softly while savouring Indian food.

|||||||||||||||||||||||||||||||||

There were many challenges in the next phase of our marriage and our personal lives. For Clair, the greatest challenge was being forced to shut down her clinical practice; such a large part of her identity had centred around her work with clients and the knowledge that she was making a difference in their lives. As for me, I learned that I could make two types of mistakes in our daily to-and-fro and give-and-take. The first type was the anxious husband reaching out to help his wife when she neither needed nor wanted assistance. The second type was my missing opportunities to help when she genuinely needed me. Type one errors were more common and really teed her off. Type two errors were mercifully less frequent—or so she said.

I comforted her when she was having a bad day, feeling irritated or frustrated. Sometimes I felt cheered up myself, reassured and relieved in being there for her. Most days we enjoyed each other, sometimes hugely. Laughing. Fighting. Making up. Making love. Teasing and joking. Snuggling. Tasting her superb rhubarb crisp. Just as in the time before Alzheimer's disease came into our lives, on our very best days we lived contentedly in the moment, in the here and now. And I was reminded of my grandmother, who would have told me, "Make hay while the sun shines!"

Learning about Alzheimer's Disease

The seeds of the book you now hold in your hands were probably planted sometime around the day that my wife and I saw the movie *Away from Her* and then shared our thoughts and feelings over dinner. But so much more has happened to her and me—and us—since that day in 2007 about which I must now write. Perhaps if I had been a little less grief-stricken, in less emotional shock over losing Clair one teaspoonful at a time, I might have done some more mental or cognitive homework back then, maybe a little more reading about what she was likely experiencing. Since that time, however, I have learned much more about this disease.

I learned, for example, from the *Global Voice on Dementia*, sponsored online by Alzheimer's Disease International, an international federation of the 75 Alzheimer associations around the world, that as of 2013 there were an estimated 44.4 million people with dementia worldwide, a number that is expected to increase to 75.6 million by 2030 and 135.5 million by 2050. There are 7.7 million new cases of dementia diagnosed each year, which means that a new case of dementia is diagnosed somewhere in the world every four seconds. According to the website, at present the cost of AD amounts to approximately 1 percent of the entire world's gross domestic product, varying from 0.24 percent of GDP in low-income countries to 0.35 percent in low middle-income countries, 0.50 percent in high middle-income countries and 1.24 percent in high-income countries. This amount is divided between that provided by family members and that provided by care professionals within the community and in care facilities, as well as the direct costs of medical care.

Variable Factors in Dementia

Although the techniques for diagnosing Alzheimer's disease have changed little over the years and are still imprecise, a diagnosis is valuable for both the patient and his/her family because a systematic assessment can eliminate other possible explanations for the symptoms a person is experiencing and the signs he/she is exhibiting. (It is useful here to note that *symptoms* are concerns, observations or complaints experienced by the patient him/herself, while *signs* are clues observed by family, friends or health care professionals. Thus, a headache is a symptom, not a sign, but memory loss to which a person is oblivious is a sign. An increased temperature that the person is aware of but that is also documented by a thermometer is both a sign and a symptom.) Recognizing early warnings and having them assessed by a family doctor are a critical first step toward diagnosis.

Warnings may include changes in memory; reasoning and judgement; speech, language and comprehension; mood and personality; and balance, gait and orientation. However, the Family Caregiver Alliance website points out that there are critical distinctions between *reversible dementias* and *irreversible dementias*. Reversible dementias result from metabolic abnormalities, endocrine imbalance, operable brain changes (hematomas, benign tumours or blood clots, for example), infections or reactions to (or interactions with) medications. Alzheimer's disease is the most frequent of the irreversible dementias, but the list also includes ischemic vascular dementia, Lewy body dementia, frontotemporal dementia, hippocampal sclerosis and Creutzfeld-Jakob dementia.

It is possible, however, for both competent family practitioners and specialists to confuse one of the treatable and reversible medical problems with a progressive dementia such as Alzheimer's, and vice versa. Hypothyroidism, for example, can slow a person down and affect his/her thinking, sometimes in a manner mimicking dementia. Anemia in older people may affect not only their energy levels but also sometimes their thought processes and memory. There is also a category within psychiatry known as the pseudodementia of depression. In this situation, a deeply depressed older person may become bedridden and lethargic, with sometimes severe cognitive slippage and memory loss. Treating that person's depression aggressively usually (although not always) results in a marked decrease in his/her depression-related cognitive and memory impairment.

While it still takes time to monitor each individual to be sure of a diagnosis, as diagnostic processes are refined and the mass of data collected in tests is analyzed, specialists are determining both more accurately and more quickly whether there is a problem, the severity of it and often the cause—or in some cases, the combination of causes. This determination helps to guide the treatment and care for the affected person and family. However, until there is a conclusive test for Alzheimer's, doctors may continue to use the phrase *probable Alzheimer's disease.*

Mild Cognitive Impairment

One step before the diagnosis of possible dementia, a doctor may refer to an individual's recent memory slippage of uncertain origin as *mild cognitive impairment,* or MCI. The Mayo Clinic website describes MCI as a stage between the memory decline that can be expected with advancing age and the memory loss typical of dementia, but MCI may affect not only memory but also language and thought processing. People with this diagnosis may repeat questions, may have difficulty performing executive functions and may struggle with mastering new job skills or organizing events. They may not notice that their mental functions have slipped because the changes may be gradual and not pronounced enough to disrupt day-to-day activities to any marked degree, but family members and close friends will be aware of changes.

Mild cognitive impairment may be accompanied by depression, irritability and aggression, anxiety or apathy. It may also be associated with the patient's risk of later progressing to dementia, but some people with mild cognitive impairment never get worse, and a few eventually get better.

Vascular Dementia

The second-most prevalent dementia after Alzheimer's disease (with or without small strokes) is vascular dementia (also known as multi-infarct dementia), which accounts for up to 20 percent of all those diagnosed. Unlike Alzheimer's disease, with its insidious onset, vascular dementia usually comes on suddenly as the result of stroke, when the blood vessels supplying oxygen to the brain become blocked or bleed, or both. Symptoms may include sudden confusion, disorientation, trouble speaking or understanding speech and loss of vision. Minor strokes, a series of transient ischemic attacks (TIAs, which raise the risk for more strokes) and other conditions that affect the smaller blood vessels may lead to cumulative brain damage, however. In such cases, cognitive symptoms may increase in a stair-step pattern; sometimes the person's abilities may deteriorate for a while, then stabilize on a plateau before deteriorating again. The person may experience gradual thinking changes, such as impaired planning and judgement, declining ability to focus, difficulty finding words and impaired function in social situations. Suspected vascular dementia can be confirmed with brain scans.

Risk factors for vascular dementia include being older than sixty-five, having high blood pressure and having a history of heart disease or diabetes. Obesity, smoking and a family history of heart problems or high cholesterol levels are additional risks. There is strong evidence, however, that the outcome can improve for the person with vascular dementia if he/she adopts a healthier lifestyle with physician-approved physical activity and a healthier diet. Reducing stress and stopping smoking can also make a big difference, as can taking medications to control high blood pressure, heart disease and diabetes.

Many people whose dementia is referred to as Alzheimer's disease also suffer from some form of vascular dementia, so that in addition to the changes in the brain that are typical of AD, the blood supply to the brain is compromised by one or more strokes. In fact, this combination of AD plus strokes is probably the most common form of dementia. That was true in Clair's case.

Lewy Body Dementia

Lewy body dementia is the third-most common type of progressive dementia. It is caused by abnormal deposits of a protein called alpha-synuclein inside the nerve cells in areas of the brain that affect thinking, memory and movement; these deposits are called *Lewy bodies* after the scientist who first described them. This type of dementia is characterized by a progressive decline in memory, language and reasoning abilities and is often associated with hallucinations. It frequently overlaps with Parkinson's disease, including the same kind of movement disorders typical of that disease, but people with Lewy bodies may also have the changes in their brains that are symptomatic of Alzheimer's and experience the same kind of cognitive slippage, sleep difficulties, mood swings and wavering attention.

Risk factors for Lewy bodies are being male, older than sixty years, and having a family member also afflicted. Obviously, these are untreatable factors.

The Diagnosis

In most cases a complete medical and neuropsychological evaluation can determine whether the person has a cognitive problem, whether it is Alzheimer's with vascular dementia (the most common presentation) or one of the other forms of dementia, and how severe it is. This will usually include the following steps.

1. A review of the patient's history, including the onset of symptoms. This information can usually be provided by a family member.

2. A medical history and list of medications. This information will include conditions that might indicate a higher risk for a particular type of dementia or identify medications that may be contributing to cognitive problems.

3. A neurological exam. This step will help to identify symptoms indicative of particular kinds of dementia or other conditions— such as stroke or Parkinson's disease—that could be increasing cognitive problems.

4. Laboratory tests to rule out vitamin deficiencies or metabolic conditions. Although not common, sometimes a simple vitamin deficiency, infection or hormone imbalance can cause cognitive symptoms.

5. A CT scan or an MRI. Brain imaging will evaluate the anatomy of the brain for conditions such as a stroke or a brain tumour that might be causing cognitive changes.

6. Mental status testing (also called cognitive or neuropsychological testing). These pencil-and-paper tests help evaluate the breadth and depth of many areas of thinking, including memory, language, problem-solving and judgement. Today the preferred screening tool is usually, although not always, the Mini-Mental Status Examination

(MMSE). However, in a pilot study with a diabetic population that was being screened for mild cognitive impairment, the Montreal Cognitive Assessment test (MoCA) appeared to be a better screening tool than the MMSE.[1]

A Checklist

If your loved one is showing signs of cognitive impairment, you can prepare for the evaluation process by doing all of the following tasks.

- Prepare a patient history, giving special attention to the onset of signs or symptoms.
- Collaborate with the patient's doctor to compile a medical history and a list of medications.
- Make an appointment for a neurological examination. (You will need your family doctor's help with this step.)
- Ask the doctor to arrange for laboratory tests to rule out vitamin deficiencies and metabolic conditions.
- Arrange for a CT scan or MRI to evaluate the anatomy of the brain. (You will also need your family doctor's help with this step.)
- Make an appointment for mental status testing.

It is widely agreed that early diagnosis of Alzheimer's disease is important to the patient. Why? Clair and I soon learned that having the diagnosis could help her move forward and gain more control over her life by taking the necessary steps to live better with the disease. The Alzheimer Society of B.C. says that early diagnosis has many benefits for patients:

- provides time to adjust to the diagnosis;
- gives an opportunity to understand the symptoms they are experiencing and the changes they can expect;
- allows them to gain access to information, resources and support;
- enables them to benefit from and explore treatment options;
- lets them play an active role in planning for their future;
- encourages them to develop and engage support networks;
- helps them maximize their quality of life.

To this list I would add that early diagnosis can bring hope and clarity to those within the marriage or partnership and allow them to have more fun. And why not? Diagnosis is prognosis, an important glimpse into the future, its threats, challenges and promises, both the negative and the positive. When you have a diagnosis, both you and your partner may anticipate a dynamic combination of grief and relief.

While no two journeys through Alzheimer's disease are alike, it may be helpful, as you find your way and make decisions for your afflicted partner, to learn how others have made the journey before you. When I asked my friend John why he had first decided to seek medical help for his wife, Nancy, he said,

> I guess I hadn't noticed anything particularly different [about her], but on reflection I can see that there was this . . . building up. But what prompted [me to take her to a doctor] was two or three episodes with the car. She had her own car and she was a good driver, but she would get lost going to pick somebody up or going to somebody's house for bridge. She'd get totally mixed up and lost. So at that point we went to our GP who was a pretty good friend as well . . . and he suggested there might be a problem. Her cholesterol was a little on the high side, so he thought she might have a vascular problem and suggested that I get her an MRI . . . and that didn't show anything. So he gave her the MMSE test [Mini Mental State Examination] and realized that there was a problem there. And then we took her to a neurologist who confirmed everything and put her on Reminyl and referred her to the UBC Alzheimer Clinic, and since then we have been going there every six months . . . they're very supportive.

For Margaret, whose husband Donald recently died from AD-related complications, the Alzheimer's diagnosis arrived like a thunderclap. He had headed up university departments, been seconded to the government to do policy work, sat on multiple boards and been headhunted to become the chief scientific officer for one of the largest technological companies in the country. When his behaviour began to change, Margaret phoned a friend at the University of BC's Brain Centre:

> He's the one who said I should bring him to the Alzheimer's clinic and have him assessed. He suggested two doctors, but we had to be referred by our family physician. There was a complete mixup, and somehow the referral got lost. So I had to go back to our family doctor a month later and do it again. By then it was 2007 so we had wasted some time. Then we went for the appointment and they ordered a CAT scan, an MRI, etcetera—you know, the usual tests—and he was diagnosed with mild cognitive impairment, and the doctor told us that 50 percent of people who

are diagnosed with MCI just go on for the rest of their lives with it. It doesn't go away, but it doesn't progress. The other 50 percent develop dementia of some type. But the following year when he went for tests, he was diagnosed with early-stage Alzheimer's.

When I asked Margaret if she and Donald had talked about the diagnosis over a drink or dinner at the time, she said,

> Do you know, I remember being in the room with him when Dr. H said to him, "Well, Donald, based on the tests I really think that you now have early-stage Alzheimer's disease," and we both sat there, just stunned. It was just a feeling of . . . you almost felt like saying, "You've made a mistake, haven't you?" But I don't remember . . . I think we talked about it when we came home, but it's blanked out. And for quite a long time after that Donald would tell people that he had mild cognitive impairment. Which was fine with me. I wasn't going to say, "No, you don't! You have Alzheimer's." You know, I thought he needs to be the one to come to terms with what this is.
>
> After that we did a clinical trial for a drug over a period of two years. It was an experimental drug and it was in Phase Two, so there was great hope because it had apparently reversed the effects of Alzheimer's in the brains of mice. So obviously there was great hope that this was what was going to happen with people. And what's interesting is that you know how, when you go into clinical trials, you don't know if you're on the drug or the placebo? Well, in my mind I was just certain that Donald was on the drug. I really did. I thought I saw an improvement. I think the mind projects things that you want, and I really thought that this was going to help him, that we could beat this like cancer or a broken arm. Well, it turned out that he was on the placebo and also that the clinical trial failed. My point is that it's strange the way your mind sees things that you want to see. I wanted to see improvement so I thought I saw improvement . . . but no . . .
>
> Donald really didn't talk too much about it. He enjoyed the process of being in the clinical trial because it gave him something to focus on, to enjoy being a scientist again . . . But he was very accepting all the way through. I mean, he was very gracious about it. I only saw him frustrated a few times and that was in the later stages when he was in the care facility . . . But really all the way through, he kept his scientific detachment. He could watch what was going on . . . He had a wonderful

analogy, you know. He said his mind was like a glacier and great chunks of memory were just falling off and floating away. Calving. It's a very powerful metaphor.

Maureen, a retired insurance broker, has been married to Merv since 1993. The first change she noticed in her husband's behaviour was his frustration with himself.

He would get really upset because of something that he would normally remember, like taxes—he had been an accountant—and he wasn't remembering. I think he was beginning to recognize that something was wrong and that frustrated him. And if I would say, "Merv, you need to do this," and if I didn't remember to say, "Would you mind?" or "I'd appreciate it if you would do this," he would get confrontational and then very angry. And I would say, "What are you angry about?" and he would answer, "I'm angry at myself. I can't stand it. I can't do anything anymore. I can't remember." Apparently he sensed the change more than I did. I noticed he was getting a little forgetful, but my goodness, we all get forgetful as we age. I took him to his doctor, and he said, "Well, he seems to have a little dementia, very mild, I guess." Merv didn't want to hear that. He said, "Dementia? You mean I'm not all right?" He got very, very upset the first time he heard those words. But after that conversation the doctor finally got through to him and put him on Aricept, but it didn't do anything for him, so I took him off that. Then it just seemed to steamroll from there.

Maureen's daughter added:

It went very fast. Just two years ago he was driving his own car and he could go to town on his own, never get lost. In the last two years the change has been just so dramatic. I guess everyone is different when it comes to this disease, but . . . well, he's so healthy! I'm concerned that he will live to be so old and just be a vegetable.

Maureen continued:

You see, he's never fallen, his legs are strong, he goes up and down steps. He's healthy, his blood pressure is perfect, his heart is perfect. It's heartbreaking. I said to him, "Well, Merv, if we could take your body and put my head on it, we'd be in great shape!" [laughter] And he might laugh, too. He had a great sense of humour and he loves to laugh. Now he makes all kinds of strange, funny noises. Even out in public.

Sometimes, of course, it is hard for a partner to recognize changes in behaviour as being the symptoms of dementia. After forty years of marriage, Graham was surprised when his wife, Yvonne, began acting strangely during a holiday in Mexico.

This happened about three or four years before she was diagnosed. It was my brother's house—a timeshare that he owned—and Yvonne and I had to sleep in the guest bedroom, and she went absolutely nuts that my brother and his wife would have the good bed and we had to sleep in the secondary bed . . . It was totally out of character. In hindsight it's my guess that was the disease beginning.

It was my sister-in-law who said, "You know, I've been reading about drugs that can assist in reducing the speed of whatever Yvonne might have, and so don't you think you should be getting her to a doctor so we can find out what it is and start getting her some treatment?" So I went to Yvonne with that argument. I'd been after her for at least two years before that, trying to get her to go to a doctor, and she just wouldn't listen. "Stop trying to run this show," she said. "Stop trying to boss me around." But she finally agreed to go, and we went to our GP who suggested we see a geriatric psychiatrist. And as soon as she saw Yvonne, she just told her what she had. It was that obvious.

I certainly was almost numb at the news. It's one of those things that you don't have any control over, you don't want to hear. You don't want to accept. Yvonne accepted it. The doctor told her she shouldn't drive a car again, and she never did from that day. She never made a fuss about it, never argued about it. I'm sure she was very upset, but I wasn't allowed to tell anybody, not even our family for ages and ages . . . And the few times that she found out that I had told somebody, she went crazy. I mean absolutely crazy. Like bizarre.

Today as soon as signs of dementia appear, our first thought is Alzheimer's disease. However, at least 20 percent of dementia patients are suffering from vascular dementia. For Sam, who had a very successful career as a logistics officer with the Royal Canadian Air Force, the process of diagnosing his dementia was very long, very slow and in the end inconclusive.

When he died in early 2015 there was still no final diagnosis, although he appeared to be suffering from vascular dementia. His problems had begun many years earlier with a diagnosis of epilepsy. In an interview in 2014 his wife, Nora, said,

> We discovered that he had epilepsy about two years after we were married. He was an RCAF pilot at that time, but he was having nocturnal seizures, so he really didn't know he was having them except that he didn't feel well the next day. Then he had a really bad one, and I saw it and insisted he get tested. So the air force threw him out—they tend to do that in the military. If you've got anything wrong with you, you're gone. But a couple of generals who knew and respected him went to bat for him; he had to change his trade to logistics, but he did very well and became a colonel.
>
> I don't think he was drinking to excess when we got married, but in those days the military encouraged the mess life and drinking because the guys were moved every two years and drinking together was a tool to make the group cohesive. Of course, they lost quite a number of good young men that way—they got really drunk and got into their fast cars and wrote themselves off. Every time that happened the military was losing thousands of dollars in training, so they're not doing so much of that anymore.

After Sam retired from the air force, he took a job with a major railroad, and that kept him in the workforce for another five years. However, at sixty-five he was forced to retire, and he and Nora settled in Calgary.

> Sam wanted to do some physical work and he had worked on a farm when he was a kid, so for three or four months each summer over the next ten years we would go to a distant cousin's ranch in central Saskatchewan and Sam would work on the harvest. He didn't work the combines but he did everything else while I would teach little kids art and work with the cousin's horses. And we were really happy up there, but then Sam began getting snarly. Yes, snarly is the only word for it. And he was starting to drink really heavily . . .
>
> I would say to my friends that he never should have retired because he was not handling it well. He didn't have any recreational interests, and he was getting more and more upset about the way his life was going. I would go off by myself to visit our daughter or

my sister and I wouldn't want to come back because he was getting more and more morose. Then about seven or eight years ago he had a small stroke and ended up in emergency. He didn't have any of the classic paralysis on one side or anything like that, but he couldn't speak. They tested him and did all the brain-wave stuff, and he must have tested out all right, but in the past four or five years he has been having small seizures while he's watching television, and he also has small absences . . . he doesn't fall down or seizure muscularly, but he's just not there . . . He's just *gone* for maybe thirty seconds or sometimes less than that.

His doctor thought he may have Parkinson's because he was going downhill on things like balance, but they decided it wasn't that. Then during the move from our old house last year he just shut totally down. He just sat in the living room of the old house with the debris all around him and sat there and sat there, and when a friend came looking for me, he stood up and fell over. So at that point people started listening to what I'd been saying. We went to the Alzheimer's clinic at UBC, and Sam took all the tests, which showed there was dementia and memory loss, but I don't think they knew what to do with him because he's not a classic case. He does very well on their pencil-and-paper tests. He scores [way] above what he should be doing—which is called showboating. The last time we went, a very nice doctor gave him another one of those visual tests, and then came out to tell me that he had done better than on his last test, so he was making improvements. Yet just that morning he had been unable to identify a picture of his grandson who has Treacher-Collins syndrome—he looks a little like a duck—and that blew me away. And he wasn't sure about identifying our other grandchildren either. So here he is supposedly doing better?

As I look back on the diagnostic doldrum days in Clair's and my own life, when it seemed as if we would never receive an answer to her worsening memory and organization problems, it seems clear that she and I had two fears: first, that we would *not* get a diagnosis, and second, that we *would* get a diagnosis. But how deadly, draconian and unacceptable would either development be to each of us, or to both of us? It's also entirely possible that her excellent physicians and neuropsychologists were experiencing some inertia or conflict as they tried to establish a diagnosis and then treat a patient who had a PhD in psychology and whose husband was—and is—an MD psychiatrist (and an anxious one at that). In any case, the doctors came through, as did the neuropsychologist who tested Clair for her problems with recent memory, judgement and problem-solving skills. Courage and competence prevailed, as they did with Clair, whom I have long experienced as both a strong and brave woman.

Then we went further. We phoned around for a second opinion and consulted with a very competent neuropsychologist in Alberta. Her findings and diagnosis of AD mirrored those shared with us in Vancouver, which came as an anticlimax and a bit more grief in our cups. But during this process, we were also given more sunlight in our overlying journeys: the sunlight of diagnosis, of focus, of clarity and of knowing where we two would be going into our shared and separate futures. Together. And apart.

If you and I were talking today—and in a way, dear reader, we are—I would want to help you recognize and appreciate the courage and strength that live in the relationship that you and your partner have worked to share, develop and enjoy over the years. And I would remind you what Clair—as well as my late wife, Betsy—have taught me, modelled for me and reminded me of supportively so many times: courage is not the absence of fear as much as it is a person's willingness and determination to push ahead in the face of fear. And with that reminder comes hope, both for the future and the present.

CHAPTER TWO

Alzheimer's Disease:
A History and an Update

For every article, paper or book published about the effects of Alzheimer's disease and other dementias on a marriage or intimate relationship, there are probably fifteen to twenty more published dealing with the effects of dementia on the larger family structure. How do we take care of Mom or Dad? How can we work together to help Grandma or Grandpa? Should we put Dad (or Mom) into a home now? Or should we put off the decision for a while longer, provided that Sis or Brother can get out here from the East Coast ASAP to look after our parent, our relative? And why does it seem that it's always *us* carrying the load for Mom's or Dad's welfare? This book does touch on and to some degree explore the effects of various dementias on the extended family, but its main emphasis is on how dementia affects the marriage, partnership or intimate relationship between two people.

First, however, it is necessary to understand more about dementia and put an end to some of the popular myths that, together with the anxiety they provoke, impede our courageous efforts to face off against the disease. We begin with Alzheimer's disease because it is now recognized as the most common type of dementia—about two of every three individuals in Canada with dementia have the AD type—and it strikes women about twice as frequently as it does men. This tragedy that today affects Clair and another thirty-six million people worldwide is growing. Its incidence is expected to double by 2030 and triple by 2050.

Alzheimer's disease, also known as Alzheimer disease or AD, was first described in a paper published in November 1906 by Dr. Alois Alzheimer, a German neuropathologist and psychiatrist. Alzheimer had been working with a patient named Auguste Deter, a woman in her early fifties who became progressively less able to care for herself at home and rejected all attempts to help her until finally she was confined in an institution that specialized in the treatment of epilepsy. When she was hospitalized, her symptoms were recorded as disorientation and impaired memory; she also had trouble reading and writing. Her symptoms gradually increased to hallucinations and an incremental loss of higher mental functions.

After her death, an investigation of her brain showed the cerebral cortex to be thinner than normal. Dr. Alzheimer noted two further abnormalities: the first was senile plaque, a structure described previously in the brains of elderly people; the second was neurofibrillary tangles—nerve tangles—in the patient's cerebral cortex. This nerve tangling had not been described previously and came to be the abnormality that helped to define the new disease. Today the diagnosis of Alzheimer's disease is still generally based on the same kind of investigative methods Alzheimer used in 1906, which is remarkable compared with the development of investigative methods for other diseases. Still, it says a lot about the quality of his discovery.

So what are these plaques and tangles? *Plaques* are deposits of amyloid-beta protein *between* the nerve cells or neurons within the brain. *Tangles* are twisted filaments of a different protein—known as the tau protein—that are found *inside* the neurons. Both develop naturally in our brains as we age, but they accumulate in much larger quantities in the brains of individuals with Alzheimer's. You can liken this process to the buildup of cobwebs, trash and garbage both outside and inside the electrical fuse box in your basement. Eventually the buildup will cause the circuits in the box to shut down one by one. But there's more. At the same time that plaques and tangles are proliferating, the synapses (the minute gaps where two nerve cells meet) and the nerve cells within the brains of AD patients become significantly fewer, and levels of acetylcholine, a neurotransmitter involved in judgement, learning and memory, are reduced.

What we still do not know is whether the plaques, the tangles and the reduction of acetylcholine in the brains of Alzheimer's patients cause Alzheimer's or are the result of Alzheimer's, or are some combination of cause and result. Think, for example, of an uncomfortably hot and humid summer day. Our experience of the temperature is not caused by the thermometer outside the kitchen door; the thermometer simply registers the temperature we are experiencing. So it may be with Alzheimer's disease.

So far, the experts seem to agree that the plaques outside the neuron bodies within the brain and the tangles within those neurons are important parts of the deadly, unrelenting progression that is Alzheimer's. There is considerably less agreement on whether one is cause and the other effect, or vice versa, or even whether both may be an expression of a process yet to be identified or named.

In his book *When the Body Says No,* physician Gabor Maté points out that among the first structures to deteriorate in Alzheimer's patients' brains are the hippocampi.[1] The hippocampi (singular hippocampus) are the twin centres of grey matter—the brain tissue responsible for transferring information between brain cells—that are located under the sides of the cerebral cortex (thus they are described as *subcortical*). Like our paired kidneys, one hippocampus can do the job if the other is ailing or non-functioning. But the job of the hippocampus is really big: it is one of the body's main memory machines, filtering new experiences before passing them on to other subcortical structures, notably the amygdalae, for storage. The functioning of the hippocampus is critical to both recent and distant memory.

Even when the hippocampus is impaired, distant memories may be recalled from the amygdala and posted there. This is why we can hang onto memories of things we learned or experienced a long time ago, such as the names of our childhood friends or the face of a favourite teacher. Recent memories, on the other hand, are much more vulnerable, as is our ability to learn new tasks. As a result, one early sign of Alzheimer's is the progressive loss of recent memory; another is the individual's inability to carry out new tasks. While most of us will exhibit these signs to a certain extent as we age, because the brain's ability to repair itself becomes steadily less efficient, it is much more pronounced for the person in the first stages of Alzheimer's. *What did I have for breakfast? Where did I park the car? With whom did I visit two days ago . . . or last week?*

Who Will Get Alzheimer's Disease?

With the founding of the Alzheimer Society of Canada in 1978, Canadian research on the origins of AD and the possibilities for prevention and cure accelerated. This society, the first of its kind in the world, was initiated after Alzheimer's researchers at the University of Toronto and Surrey Place Centre became deeply concerned about the lack of support available to families affected by the disease. A steering group composed of researchers, family members, professional staff and a resource person was formed, and while the new organization did provide more support for families caring for loved ones with this disease, the Society's primary goal soon became research.

By the 1990s teams of scientists, with Canadians playing central roles, were focusing on investigating whether there were genetic links in Alzheimer's disease, using mouse models that made it possible to do research that had previously been impractical. By 1992 they had confirmed that in a small percentage of familial AD cases, a mutated gene predisposed family members to AD. The big question then became how important and how prevalent genetic factors are in causing Alzheimer's disease.

Scientists have now discovered that both deterministic and risk genes can be involved in the development of AD. *Deterministic genes*—those genes that *guarantee* anyone inheriting them will develop a particular disorder—can be the direct cause of AD, but deterministic Alzheimer's variations have been found in only a few hundred extended families world-wide. On the other hand, several *risk genes* implicated in AD—that is, genes that *increase the likelihood* of developing the disease but don't guarantee it will happen—have been identified. It is estimated that the risk gene with the strongest influence, known as APOE-e4, could be a factor in 20 to 25 percent of AD cases. If an individual inherits APOE-e4 from one parent, he/she is at an increased risk of Alzheimer's; if the individual inherits the gene from both parents, the risk is even higher. It is important to understand, however, that development of the disease is still not a certainty. In addition, the symptoms for someone carrying this risk factor tend to appear at an earlier age—as young as thirty or forty. However, this early-onset type of AD is very rare, affecting less than five percent of people who develop AD. We now also know that the disease in this early-onset form often has multiple genetic components linked to it, and they are often interwoven in complex ways.

In a 2014 article, C.T. Loy et al. explain that just 25 percent of people over the age of fifty-five who are diagnosed with AD have a family history of dementia.[2] Within the families of this 25 percent, however, there are many small genetic "deviations" so that family members' lifetime risk of dementia increases to about 20 percent, compared to a 10 percent lifetime risk in the general population.

More Information about Risk

According to the Alzheimer Society of Canada website, "The sporadic form of Alzheimer's disease, which used to be called late onset Alzheimer's disease, was formerly assumed to have no family linkages. However, it's now known that a person with a direct relative (parent or sibling) with Alzheimer's disease has a three times greater chance of developing the disease than someone who does not. The risk increases if both parents have the disease." The website then provides this risk formula: "Of 100 people with no defined genetic risk factor, five will get Alzheimer's disease at age 65 or older (and 95 will not). Of 100 people, each with a parent with Alzheimer's disease, 15 will get Alzheimer's at age 65 or older (and 85 will not)."

The Nun Study

One of the most interesting probes into the possible causes and early signs of Alzheimer's is the Nun Study.[3] Begun in 1986, this longitudinal study, the product of research initiated by scientist David Snowdon, continues to widen and deepen our understanding of the disease today. Dr. Snowdon has been studying 678 members of the School Sisters of Notre Dame religious congregation, delving into their personal and medical histories, testing them for cognitive function and even dissecting their brains after death. These nuns had relatively homogeneous backgrounds, including no drug use, little or no alcohol consumption, similar educational backgrounds and similar housing and reproductive histories, that help control for extraneous variables in the study.

The results of Snowdon's work have added volumes to our knowledge of the disease. For example, his review of autobiographical essays written by the nuns upon joining the sisterhood at an average age of twenty-two showed that an essay's lack of linguistic density or complexity was a significant predictor of the writer's risk for developing Alzheimer's disease in old age. In fact, roughly 80 percent of the nuns whose early writing lacked complexity went on to develop Alzheimer's disease in old age; of those whose writing was not lacking in this complexity, only 10 percent later developed the disease. His findings also showed that those nuns who expressed more positive emotions within their early writings lived significantly longer, and those struggling with AD experienced fewer positive emotions as their Alzheimer's progressed.

Snowdon's study supports the ideas that reading and keeping intellectually busy, avoiding head injuries and strokes and taking certain nutritional supplements such as folic acid and antioxidants can be beneficial in avoiding Alzheimer's disease. However, even more interesting is his discovery at autopsy that some of the women—for example, the Mother Superior—had brain changes consistent with Alzheimer's despite that they were extremely competent right to the end of their days.

The Long Goodbye

Former US President Ronald Reagan was officially diagnosed with Alzheimer's Disease in 1994, five years after he left the White

House. He died of pneumonia complicated by Alzheimer's ten years later, on June 5, 2004. His wife, Nancy Reagan, described the disease that afflicted her husband as "The Long Goodbye." She attributed the onset of Alzheimer's to a riding accident a few months after Reagan left office (he suffered a concussion and a subdural hematoma in the fall) and insists he was free of Alzheimer's symptoms while he was in office. Others, however, have cited instances of his confusion and his inability to remember people and names in the last years of his presidency. The medical community has been unable to prove conclusively that acute brain injury accelerates Alzheimer's disease or any other form of dementia.

The 90+ Study

Led by Dr. Claudia Kawas, a geriatric neurologist, and Maria Corrada, an epidemiologist, the ground-breaking 90+ Study is now in its second decade.[4] The work is based at the Clinic for Aging Research and Education in the former retirement community of Leisure World, now incorporated as the city of Laguna Woods, California. The researchers are seeking answers to questions such as what makes people live to ninety and beyond, what kinds of food and lifestyles are associated with living longer and what enables people to remain dementia free into their nineties. The fourteen thousand participants are visited every six months by neuropsychological testers and neurological examiners to obtain information on diet, activities, medical history and medications, and are given cognitive and physical tests to determine function. The results of this study are gradually being made available to researchers around the world, but the study has already produced startling information. For instance, researchers have learned that people who drink moderate amounts of coffee or alcohol live longer than abstainers, and that people who are overweight in their seventies live longer than normal-weight or underweight individuals. They have also discovered that more than 40 percent of people ninety or older suffer from dementia, while almost 80 percent are physically disabled (both conditions are more common in women than in men). About half of the people over ninety who are living with dementia don't have sufficient Alzheimer's-related plaque growth in their brains to explain their cognitive loss. Individuals aged ninety or older who carry the APOE2 gene are less likely to have Alzheimer's-like dementia but are much more likely to have Alzheimer's-related plaque growth in their brains. Notably, the researchers have found that poor performance on activities such as walking is indicative of increased risk of dementia.

A Lifestyle Disease

Like the 90+ Study, other research suggests that Alzheimer's is primarily a lifestyle disease, and several studies have posited correlations between various cardiovascular risk factors (high cholesterol, high blood pressure, diabetes and smoking) and increased risk of Alzheimer's. Earlier studies had already suggested that adhering to a Mediterranean-style diet—that is, one centred on vegetables, fruits, fish, whole grains, nuts, olive oil and a moderate amount of alcohol, with a limited consumption of red meat, refined sugar and refined grains—is associated with a lower risk of heart disease, stroke and cognitive disorders like Alzheimer's disease.

In 2012 a study led by researchers at the University of Miami and Columbia University went one step further, and the results suggest that the Mediterranean diet might actually protect against blood damage in the brain, thus reducing the risk of stroke and memory loss.[5] In this study nearly one thousand people were asked to fill in food questionnaires; participants were then grouped according to how closely they adhered to the ideal Mediterranean-style diet. Participants then underwent magnetic resonance imaging (MRI) to discover white matter hyperintensities, which indicate the small blood vessel damage that can cause so-called silent strokes. These strokes have no immediate outward symptoms, but over time can affect cognitive performance. The results showed that people with the highest Mediterranean diet scores had the lowest white-matter volume burden. But the researchers also found that those who consumed more monounsaturated fat, such as that found in olive oil, had lower white-matter hyperintensity volumes on their brain scans. While the study doesn't prove that eating a Mediterranean-style diet will mean less brain damage, it does suggest that the diet might protect the small blood vessels in the brain.

Obesity, diabetes and metabolic syndrome (which includes high blood pressure, high blood-sugar levels, excess fat around the waist and abnormal cholesterol levels) are all increasingly common in North America and are primary risk factors in the most common form of dementia. Noting this point, researchers at the University of Cincinnati were able to show that what matters most is how individuals superimpose their lifestyles on their genetic background.[6] Their study found, for example, that carbohydrate restriction helped participants who had mild cognitive impairment, which is often associated with early Alzheimer's, to regain mental function.

Meanwhile, other brain experts agree on the merits of a diet high in proteins and rich in colourful fruits and vegetables as the latter are strong in polyphenols and antioxidants, which have been proven to boost brain health. Long-term use of non-steroidal anti-inflammatory drugs (NSAIDs), drinking three to five cups of coffee per day at midlife, engaging in intellectual activities (reading, playing board games, crossword puzzles, playing musical instruments) and regular social interaction are all associated with a reduced likelihood of developing AD. Some authorities have also suggested that medical marijuana may be effective in inhibiting the progress of AD. Thus, it appears that even if you do carry a genetic predisposition, lifestyle modifications in mid-life can greatly reduce your risk of Alzheimer's or other forms of dementia, or at least delay their onset.

Ginger for Preventing Dementia?

University of British Columbia neurologist Dr. Patrick McGeer has, with his wife, Dr. Edith McGeer, spent a lifetime researching the degenerative neurological diseases of aging. In February 2012 he told a conference of the American Association for the Advancement of Science that in his own small lab study, using mice that had been genetically altered to give them Alzheimer-like pathology, he had been able to demonstrate that ginger extract cleared amyloid-beta aggregations from brains riddled with it, thereby helping to prevent buildup of protein plaque.[7] As a result, the eighty-four-year-old said, he now ate ginger every day as one of his personal strategies for warding off Alzheimer's disease. He also recommended that people eat blackberries, rhubarb, cinnamon, turmeric, cranberries, pomegranates and blueberries, all of which contain enzymes that prevent plaque buildup.

McGeer then suggested that agents to prevent plaque buildup might be found in drugs that are already in use for other applications, while some preventive agents may be found in the components of herbal medicines. However, because herbal medicines are cheap, there is a strong disincentive for pharmaceutical companies to embark on high-cost clinical trials to prove their value in treating dementia.

Coconut Oil for Preventing Dementia?

Berkeley Wellness, a publication of the University of California Berkeley, reports that Dr. Mary Newport, attempting to halt her Alzheimer's-afflicted husband's decline, was impressed by research suggesting that increasing ketones (by-products of the breakdown of fats in the body) may improve outcomes in various neurological disorders.[8] One of the ways to boost ketone levels is the consumption of medium-chain triglycerides (MCTs), which are converted in the liver into ketones; the brain and other organs can then use them as immediate fuel because they provide energy to cells without the need for insulin, the hormone the body normally relies on to get glucose from the blood into the cells.

Both coconut and palm kernel oils are good sources of MCT. Dr. Newport chose to feed to her husband coconut oil, later combining it with another, more concentrated MCT oil. She reported that his short-term memory improved, his depression lifted, his personality revived and his vision and walking problems were reduced. An MRI showed that his brain had stopped shrinking. Dr. Newport's reported results are, however, totally subjective and entirely anecdotal. Her husband's long-term outcome remains unknown because the course of Alzheimer's disease varies from patient to patient, with stable periods and temporary improvement windows appearing within the overall decline.

Meanwhile, new research has shown that stress is an important factor to watch and monitor in Alzheimer's and other dementias. Scientists in a recent study at Yale found that stressful events—such as job loss or death of a loved one—appeared to cause the brain's grey matter to shrink, leading to cognitive impairment.[9] But interestingly, the authors found that in instances where stress is dealt with in a healthy manner—exercising, cultivating positive personal relationships and engaging in wholesome activities—dendrites (which transfer information between brain cells) will grow back.

Stress raises the body's level of cortisol, a hormone that increases blood glucose, which in turn increases insulin. Dr. Ira Goodman of Orlando Health told the *Orlando Sentinel* that, "We believe . . . the impaired ability to use or make insulin contributes to neurodegeneration—in other words, brain breakdown. Eating fewer carbohydrates helps keep insulin levels down."[10] He notes further that "if it's good for your heart, it's good for your brain."

People who have taken statins for years to control their cholesterol levels seem to have protection from the buildup of plaques and tangles, as do those who keep their blood pressure down with or without medication. Anti-inflammatory medications also help. For example, those who developed arthritis early in life and began taking NSAIDs are at lower risk of developing Alzheimer's. Exercising your body and your brain is a protective strategy. Dr. Ira Goodman notes,

> The more you learn, the more synapses you make. Brain degeneration involves the breaking down of synapses, so the more you have, the longer the brain takes to break down. This is why we think people who are highly educated have a lower incidence of Alzheimer's.[11]

Researchers have also found that socializing with friends and actively practising a faith can help. And, although the relationship between bilingualism and cognition is very complicated, several studies indicate that bilingualism delays the onset of Alzheimer's disease. For example, a 2013 study reviewed records of 648 dementia patients, more than half of whom were bilingual.[12] The researchers looked at the age at which symptoms were first manifest and found that dementia developed on average 4.5 years later in bilingual patients than in patients who spoke only one language. They also discovered that this outcome was consistent even with bilingual patients who were illiterate, suggesting that education was not a factor in the findings. Interestingly, the researchers found no additional benefit to speaking more than two languages. The jury is still out on *why* bilingualism seems to delay Alzheimer's onset, but research is ongoing.

And what about the statistics that say twice as many women as men get Alzheimer's disease? Some researchers believe this to be the result of women's hormonal changes at menopause, in particular the decline of the hormone estrogen, which may protect the brain from age-related changes that could lead to cognitive impairment and dementia. The risk may be increased for women who have had hysterectomies and complete removal of the ovaries, bringing on premature menopause. Another factor in this imbalance may be that women are more prone to diabetes, which also appears to be a risk factor for the onset of Alzheimer's disease. Recently a gene has been identified that occurs only in women and appears to increase the risk for Alzheimer's slightly. However, the preponderance of women with the disease and the fact that more women than men are living out their final years in care homes may simply be the result of women living longer than men—by an average of six years in high-income countries and three years in low-income countries.

The final risk factor for developing Alzheimer's—one that many of us probably have mixed feelings about—is aging. Unfortunately, this is one factor over which we have no control.

Diagnosing the Disease

Improvement in diagnostic techniques for Alzheimer's disease has been slow but modestly encouraging. Recent research using positron emission tomography (PET), for example, has helped confirm the speculation that the plaques within the brain that are associated with Alzheimer's—and confirmed at autopsy—could be present as much as ten to fifteen years before actual clinical presentation.[13] In addition, Bateman et al. report that certain genetic types of Alzheimer's have demonstrated that biomarkers for the disease, such as tau levels, may increase as much as fifteen years before the expected onset of symptoms.[14] More recently, Tom Valeo reported that other biomarkers have been found in cerebrospinal fluid (CSF) obtained by lumbar punctures (spinal taps).[15] A decrease in amyloid-beta plaque within the CSF suggests a corresponding increase in protein fragments, which are the biomarkers within the brain. There is also a growing consensus that PET imaging can now be used to identify subjects with elevated plaque levels even at the early pre-clinical stages of the disease.

Meanwhile, a study out of the University of Rochester Medical Center has described the successful search for and validation of ten lipids that predicted conversion to either symptomatic mild cognitive impairment or Alzheimer's within a two- to three-year period.[16] The procedure provides 90 percent accuracy in diagnosing a cognitively normal elderly population of subjects. However, implementation of this procedure among the general population remains distant.

Arresting or Reversing Alzheimer's Disease

While methods to predict dementias continue to improve and strategies for preventing dementia proliferate, the most frequent question among laypeople is when research will find the means to arrest and reverse the dreadful dementia a loved one is struggling with. The answer coming from researchers is "Soon . . . we hope."

The initial line of inquiry for early Alzheimer's researchers was tracking the function of acetylcholine, a neurotransmitter involved in judgement, learning and memory. By 1997 the pharmaceutical companies Eisai and Pfizer, working together, had developed and received approval for the cholinesterase inhibitor Aricept, the first drug for treating Alzheimer's disease. It worked by blocking the activity of cholinesterase, an enzyme that breaks down acetylcholine and helped to reduce the symptoms of mild to moderate Alzheimer's in some individuals. Its success was followed within five years by two more drugs offering treatment alternatives that help to slow, although not stop, AD symptoms for six to twelve months.

In 2004 pharmaceutical company Eli Lilly released Memantine, an "NMDA receptor blocker" to stabilize or slow the decline of cognitive function in people with moderate to advanced Alzheimer's. Memantine works by binding to specific brain receptor cells and blocking the activity of the neurotransmitter glutamate; at normal levels, glutamate aids in memory and learning, but if levels are too high, as happens in Alzheimer's, it appears to overstimulate nerve cells, killing them through over-activity and causing cognitive defects. When this drug was given to Clair, her Alzheimer's showed modest improvement (for a while she was more focused or attentive), but it was discontinued when staff at her care centre felt that negative behaviour changes—including aggressiveness—outweighed any positive change.

Each new piece of knowledge that researchers establish leads science closer to the whole picture, however. For example, some recent biochemical studies of people with and without Alzheimer's disease have focused on the brain mechanisms that protect against neuro-degeneration. In 2014 researcher Tao Lu and colleagues at Harvard University found a factor that appears to protect brain functioning within the cerebral and hippocampal cortex.[17] By repressing destructive genes that facilitate both cell death and Alzheimer's, the RE1-Silencing Transcription factor (REST) acts to encourage genes that combat oxidative stress. They also found that REST is diminished or lost in mild cognitive impairment, Alzheimer's, frontotemporal and Lewy body dementias, and its absence or loss correlated with the pathological misfolding of brain proteins. They concluded that REST levels in the course of aging are closely correlated with cognitive preservation and longevity.

The very newest theories and hypotheses into the causes of Alzheimer's are leading researchers in a wide variety of directions. The cholinergic hypothesis suggests that AD is caused by reduced production of the neurotransmitter acetylcholine, a compound that transmits impulses from nerve fibres. Therefore, many pharmaceutical companies are trying to design AD medicines that increase acetylcholine production to slow AD in its earliest phases; unfortunately, none of these medicines have proved helpful in the later stages of AD. Both the cholinergic hypothesis and a newer amyloid hypothesis (which focuses on finding ways to break down the amyloid beta deposits within the brain) have been recently upstaged, to some extent, by a tau hypothesis. This hypothesis focuses on tau protein abnormalities that form neurofibrillary tangles inside the nerve cell bodies, destroying the cells from the inside out.

Following the Amyloid Plaque Trail

There seemed to be good news in July 2015 when the *Guardian* newspaper published an article entitled "Scientists find first drug that appears to slow Alzheimer's disease."[18] The story reported that trials of a drug called Solanezumab, developed by Eli Lilly, had been shown to slow memory loss in patients with mild Alzheimer's disease by causing the plaques in the brain to disintegrate. Although an eighteen-month trial of the drug on a large group of patients with both mild and moderate dementia—half taking the drug and half on a placebo—had appeared to end in failure in 2012, a more thorough analysis of the data showed that, among the 1,300 patients within the test group who had only mild Alzheimer's, those on the drug had showed a roughly 30 percent slower decline in memory and cognitive tests than those who had taken the placebo. As this hinted that the drug could help as long as it was taken early enough, those taking the placebo were put on the drug as well and the trial continued for another two years. According to the *Guardian* story, it was felt that if the drug had just been treating the symptoms of AD, the group taking the placebo would have caught up with the others when they started taking the drug as well. However, after two years there were still differences between them, so it was concluded that the drug must have made inroads on the disease, not just the symptoms. In November 2016, however, after Phase 3 trials of the drug were concluded, Eli Lilly announced that patients treated with Solanezumab had not experienced statistically significant slowing of cognitive decline, and the company was abandoning future trials.

But all of these hypotheses are still just guesses—educated guesses, to be sure, but not definitive answers and certainly not cures. Answers have been—and probably will be for a while longer—harder to come by. In the meantime, the research landscape has become highly personalized, even politicized, with different research chemists, physicians and neuropathologists approaching cause-and-effect questions from very different perspectives. Pharmaceutical companies are observing all this research and betting on their own medications from a host of different perspectives. In 2009 Andrea Gillies wrote an excellent summary of the tensions within the Alzheimer's research community, noting that

> Pro-tau scientists have had enormous trouble getting research grants or getting their results published in medical journals [because] the plaque orthodoxy has become quite medieval in its tolerance of heretics. So it's heartening to see that the latest wonder drug, Rember, is a tau-directed one. Perhaps the orthodoxy is being challenged now.[19]

Arresting or Reversing Decline

Dale E. Bredesen, the director of Neurogenerative Disease Research at the David Geffen School of Medicine at UCLA, led a group of researchers who conducted a novel therapeutic program using individual plans to correct body imbalances for a select group of ten individuals.[20] All suffered from some form of cognitive decline: memory loss associated with Alzheimer's, amnestic mild cognitive impairment (aMCI) or subjective cognitive impairment (SCI). All of the individualized patient programs included dietary and lifestyle changes as well as supplements. For example, most patient protocols included eliminating simple carbohydrates, gluten and processed food from the diet while increasing vegetables, fruit and non-farmed fish; exercising a minimum of thirty minutes per day; and practising yoga and meditation to relieve stress. Patients also took herbs such as *Bacopa monnieri*, ashwagandha and turmeric, and supplements such as melatonin, methylcobalamin, methyltetrahydrofolate, citicoline, vitamins D3, C and E, CoQ10 and DHA (docosahexaenoic acid), coconut oil and fish oil.

Of the five women and five men in the program, six had been forced to stop working or were struggling to function in the workplace; after a few months in the program, all six were again able to perform effectively at work. Three more made definite improvement and now function normally in society. The tenth subject entered the program when she was already in the middle stages of Alzheimer's, and continued to decline despite her individualized regimen. These results appeared to indicate that the program could reverse or improve memory loss in patients with subjective cognitive impairment, mild cognitive impairment and the early stage of Alzheimer's disease, although Dr. Bredesen noted that his team's results were anecdotal, and a more extensive controlled clinical trial was needed.

He also concedes that this program is not easy. None of the ten patients followed the entire protocol, the diet and lifestyle changes and multiple daily doses of pills being their most common complaints. But he sees a potentially important application of his program as a platform on which drugs that would fail as "monotherapeutics," or individual treatments, might succeed as key components in a multi-therapy system. Combination therapies have proven successful in illnesses such as HIV and cancer.

In the meantime, well-documented research competes with anecdotal reports (such as "I have an aunt in Iowa with Alzheimer's who took salmon oil, and now she's a hundred percent better!"). Reports from popular media may complement, support or contradict rigorously controlled research projects from the scientific community. Whom should we believe? People want answers, especially when the disease strikes close to home. And the closer it comes, the more quickly, eagerly and at times impulsively and uncritically we will reach out for chancy, unsafe and uncertain theories and conclusions offered by unproven sources.

By all means, listen to your friends' experiences and follow the latest medical news, but do so with caution. We must be careful, very careful, with anecdotal reports. It is much better not to hope for quick fixes and to be surprised when they happen than the opposite. Instead, remember that your doctor usually has the most up-to-date information, and he/she may refer you to a geriatric psychiatrist whose business it is to know what is happening in the field. Meanwhile, enjoy your partner and his/her warmth while you can, while your loved one is here with you. Make hay while the sun shines.

CHAPTER THREE

Finding Help and Comfort
for Your AD Partner

After Clair's Alzheimer's diagnosis was relayed to us on that cool spring day in 2007, we called a family meeting in our apartment to announce the news, and then together—all of us except my own kids in Oregon—we shared and listened quietly. Clair's words of comfort for us were warm, straightforward, gracious and full of courage. "We've got a slight problem here—it'll probably be a challenge—so let's stick together and keep an eye on each other!" was what she seemed to be saying that night.

About nine or ten months later I arranged a second family meeting, this time overseen by my therapist, Molly, and without Clair's participation. It was less warm, more tense and anxious, as everyone had difficulty sharing what they were experiencing: the persistent and progressive loss of my wife and my step-kids' mother. Why the change in tenor between the two meetings when they were less than a year apart? I'm not sure, except that everyone—save myself—was a stranger to Molly and her office. Sharing grief, loss, anger and frustration in these circumstances may have been difficult for most of us—perhaps all of us. But this session was followed by a meeting with Clair in my office that gave us another chance to unload more with counsellors, therapists and psychologists, all of whom enjoyed enormous mutual respect with Clair. She reflected on her bad news with humour. After that meeting there were tears mixed with hugs, silences and notes of quietly shared cheer and support.

|||||||||||||||||||||||||||||||||

In my practice as a psychotherapist I have found that the statement "I need help!" is most often and most easily answered with the question "For whom?" If you're like most of us with a partner suffering from AD, you are probably focusing fully on your partner while secretly telling yourself, "I'll take care of me later when it's quiet or when I have time or . . ." So first let's follow your likely thought processes and sequencing to give you some support and ideas for getting help for your partner.

At this point you have your partner's diagnosis, and she/he is probably still living at home with you. Is this arrangement working out to your mutual satisfaction? Do you have a solid, kind, sensitive and competent family practitioner who is comfortable with being there for each of you, and for both of you, at this time? In Nora's case, although she and her husband have different doctors, the doctors are colleagues. When I suggested that it might work better if they had the same doctor, Nora said,

> Except that I've had the same doctor for so long and I trust her. She saved me by recognizing that I had temporal arteritis [in 2011]. And when I brought up that problem [of having different doctors] to her, she just said, "When the time comes, Nora, we [she and Sam's doctor] will work in tandem." And they handled him very well together when he was in hospital with an infection, and he had one of his outbursts. He was really a handful.

At this time caregivers should also be looking for a support group, either formal or informal, for the patient.

"Alzheimer cafes put the focus on the person," read the headline on one news story.[1] The staff at the Ridgewood Veterans Wing of the Saint John Regional Hospital were about to host the province's first Alzheimer café, a place for people with dementia and their families to meet for coffee and listen to an expert speak about the effects of the disease. At that time approximately ten thousand people in the Saint John area were in some way affected by Alzheimer's disease. Ed Sullivan, the seventy-year-old organizer, felt that if the disease were discussed openly in a café-like forum, the person, rather than the disease, would be the focus.

I'm not sure Clair, who by that time was moving steadily into the middle stages of Alzheimer's, would have enjoyed sitting around listening to an expert speak about the disease. For that matter, I'm not sure I would have either, but for caregivers and/or those in the early onset stages of AD, events of this kind can be very helpful and may provide a welcome opportunity to socialize.

Our local Alzheimer's Association sponsors several groups for people with mild to moderate AD and their caregiving spouses, and here the sharing of frustrations, loneliness and other overlapping themes, as well as conflicts and laughter, can be quite comforting for all involved. Clair and I tried one of these groups briefly, but she was put off by the bibs provided at the lunches that were sponsored by the support group and refused to go back. Nothing ventured, nothing gained. However, Margaret's husband, Donald, did find support at an adult daycare centre. She told me,

> At first I thought, well, he's never been a joiner, he was always very much a loner, but he went there and he really enjoyed it. He thoroughly enjoyed it, and I think it was because he felt comfortable with everyone else. I mean, there were other people there who had minor cognitive impairment or Alzheimer's or whatever, and he found some really good buddies there. One fellow didn't have Alzheimer's but he was very frail, and they asked him to go to the centre so he could make some social connections, and he and Donald became good friends because Donald could follow along. Although he'd lost some of his memories, a lot of his cognitive abilities remained. I think the daycare experience gave him a lot of support and it gave me support because he went Mondays and Fridays and it gave me some freedom to get out as well.

Although the dementia that Nora's husband, Sam, suffers from is not diagnosed as Alzheimer's, her doctor directed her to a support group run by the Alzheimer's Society. There are six or seven couples in this group, and two of the "memory loss" people in it are dealing with vascular dementia rather than AD. Nora explained:

> I was very surprised how many men caregivers there are in the group, and they are really good caregivers from what I can see. These are sterling guys. We use the gym for an hour every Friday, exercising on chairs because some of the memory loss people have balance problems. There's a trainer who runs the session and always two volunteers who sit beside the people who are having the most problems. I don't sit beside Sam because I have a tendency to nag, and I've noticed that the guys who were sitting beside their wives telling them what to do are not doing that anymore. They sit across from them now. After working out on chairs we play a game, and they try to get us up dancing. Sam can't dance. He's lost that . . . even to walk forward is difficult for him, but to walk backward or shuffle sideways—even holding on

to me—is too much for him. He's lost that coordination. In the second hour we go to the community room and play word games in groups of three or four with the caregivers separated from the memory loss people—and often they do better than we do! [laughter] Like the lady who used to run a bookstore before she had AD, she can ace anything in that field, and Sam can still ace anything to do with planes.

A good diet, plenty of exercise (remember: if it's good for the heart, it's good for the head), intellectual stimulation and socialization are all pieces to this puzzle of how to help your husband, wife or partner enjoy the time he/she has today. As well as the afternoon daycare program, Margaret found one-on-one socialization for her husband in an unlikely source.

We had a cleaning lady, and one day she announced that she was retiring—she was going to stop cleaning—and suddenly a light bulb went on in my head. She and Donald would often talk and they got along really well, so I phoned her and said, "Would you like to come over and spend some time with Donald? You know, three or four hours, take him out for walks or just talk with him?" And she said, "Sure." And so that worked out fine, and she was also a former cook, so she could cook things for him as well.

In the first twelve to eighteen months following her diagnosis, Clair and I pretty much lived in the here and now. Maybe we were doing some of that before, I don't know, but afterwards we certainly made hay while the sun shone. We fought and made up. Made love. Laughed together and apart. Had fun. Visited our children and grandchildren. Cooked for ourselves and for each other. Clair loved to read, especially short stories, and it seemed to be a treat for her to snuggle with me at night while she consumed the latest and best articles and short stories in the *New Yorker*. I know it was a treat for me.

Also, don't put travelling off until tomorrow. Clair and I took several trips shortly before her diagnosis was clear. One was to Scotland, a memorable trip that was overseen and coordinated by my brother, Douglas. He drove, narrating with his lovely, supportive wife, Terrie, while in the back seat Clair and I enjoyed the view, the sights and especially the narrative. We were treated like royalty! A second trip saw us visiting Israel with twenty members of our Synagogue Har El, a trip that was conducted by a super, fluently bilingual travel guide. Neither of these trips would have been possible later; so the moral is, live in the moment where you are and where you can be. We also visited friends and family in Oregon, Washington and the Netherlands and attended several professional meetings that we were both able to enjoy (along with the socialization and fun that so often accompany such events). Clair's family accompanied me on the STP—the two-day Seattle-to-Portland bike race—two years in a row (2008 and 2009), and Clair went with them as part of my "road crew." I am so grateful for those memories today.

At home we continued to entertain both local and out-of-town friends and family, and I am so glad now that we took advantage of those opportunities when we did. Those same family and friends appreciated the chance to be with both of us when Clair was still at her very best—or close to it. It was enjoyment all the way around.

Cooking for yourselves and each other may be important for both of you. While you're at it, why not have a discussion over dinner some night—or nights—about your partner's wishes for the future? What does she/he dream of doing? What are her/his hopes? Fears? Fantasies? Conflicts? Don't forget to share your own thoughts and fantasies. My main point here is to encourage each of you—and both of you—to continue on normal pathways together and separately as long as possible.

For twelve to eighteen months after the diagnosis, Clair visited my counsellor, Molly, with me, and we were both able to share dreams, hopes, fears, agreements and disagreements. However, as her AD progressed, Clair was not the active participant she had been before, and eventually the time came when she would wait upstairs for me while I shared my hopes and fears, my dreams and fantasies and moments of anxiety with Molly alone.

||||||||||||||||||||||||||||||||||||

The professional literature on Alzheimer's disease is sterner and less emotional than most of us are prepared for. Fuelled by a tankful of tough love, it tells it like it is. But some of it can be extraordinarily helpful for those of us, especially family and close friends, who are facing such a loss; often the stern tone is even comforting. One day, for example, while browsing in my home library, I came across the book *The Alzheimer's Action Plan: What You Need to Know—and What You Can Do—About Memory Problems from Prevention to Early Intervention and Care.* I noticed that it contained one of Clair's Visa receipts from our local bookstore dated July 2009, almost two and a half years after we had finally obtained a diagnosis. Interestingly, a section of this book entitled "Our Top 40 Questions and Answers" addressed two questions that Clair had been struggling with right around the time she bought the book.

One question came from a husband in his sixties whose wife had early-onset Alzheimer's. He wanted to know how she could complain about having nothing to do yet not get any of the housework done. The book's authors explained how people with Alzheimer's gradually lose their executive function—that is, the ability to plan, organize and then carry out a process, even a simple thing like getting dressed. In the early stages of the disease, it may be enough to leave notes and phone reminders to help the person stay organized, but as the effects of the disease increase, AD partners will need someone, such as a paid companion, to keep them on track.

Like the wife of the man who posed the question, in the summer of 2009 Clair had been complaining that she had been "doing all the work around here for some time now!" My own memory of that time was of her being peeved whenever I did venture to help around the house. And how did I respond as we struggled with two such different Alzheimer experiences? I learned never to argue with her.

Another question the authors dealt with concerned the fact that many people with Alzheimer's make up stories, especially when it comes to sexual affairs, often accusing their partners of being involved with someone else. This was also a problem Clair and I had been having around that time, although from a different point of view. She wasn't worried about me seeing someone else. Her anxious misunderstanding was that she and I were having an affair and that "David might find out." This thought upset her so much that one evening we had to excuse ourselves halfway through our yoga class because she was worried that David might discover us there. She also accompanied me to southern Oregon to visit my own kids but wondered out loud somewhere between Eugene and Ashland, Oregon, what we would do "if David finds out about us?"

"He's a big boy—I bet he can take care of himself!" I guessed out loud.

The *Alzheimer's Action Plan* authors' response to this question is that the two most common delusions of people with dementia concern imagined infidelity and theft by family members. The first of these problems—imagined infidelity—probably arises from a deep-rooted fear of abandonment in a world that has become strange and confusing, and no amount of logical argument is going to wipe away that fear. In any case, arguing is likely to be misinterpreted as anger, which will exacerbate the situation. Instead, the answer for the caregiving partner is quiet reassurance that he/she will always be there. Now, looking back on the uncertain moments that Clair and I had shared at that time, I could appreciate that what she had worried about had made a certain kind of sense—except she wasn't having an affair with another man. Instead, *I* was having an affair with another woman: the woman Clair was becoming.

People with the initial signs and symptoms of Alzheimer's disease frequently experience anxiety, although as the AD progresses, the victim's anxiety is often, though not always, observed to lessen. The most common anxiety triggers are unfamiliar objects (e.g., new furniture or clothes), people (e.g., different caregivers or unfamiliar people in the home) and situations (e.g., a change in environment) as well as expectations to perform (e.g., to answer a question). In response to a challenge to perform, an AD patient might exhibit anxiety of such magnitude that it must be described as catastrophic, not unlike a panic attack. Dr. Gene D. Cohen, founding director of the Center on Aging, Health and Humanities at George Washington University, explained that anxiety can even occur in familiar surroundings if the AD patient is disengaged or isolated there; he likens this to the separation anxiety some young children experience when placed in an unfamiliar environment.[2] Since both the very young and the AD patient have a limited capacity to explain what they are feeling, he suggests, it is instead up to the caregiver to interpret what the patient is displaying.

Such catastrophic reactions in AD patients can often be resolved by distracting them in the same way that one handles a temper tantrum in a two-year-old; in fact, the central nervous system phenomena operating in both situations may be related. As with the two-year-old, when an AD patient displays anxiety in such situations, it may be enough to simply alter the experience to reassure the patient. When the patient is returned to a familiar setting or is among familiar faces, the anxiety will often disappear quickly.

There is one more problem facing spouses who elect to keep their partners with newly diagnosed AD at home: wandering. According to the Alzheimer's Association's national database, 60 percent of people in the earliest stages of AD will wander, becoming disoriented and lost even in their own familiar neighbourhoods. As they generally don't know how to ask for assistance or directions, most are unable to return home, and if not found within twenty-four hours, up to half of these wanderers will suffer serious injury or death. Some wanderers are attempting to return to a half-remembered location, trying to go to a job they once held or to go home from work when they are already home. Others are trying to escape from stress or noise. Sometimes they are simply searching for something to eat or drink, or for the bathroom, and have forgotten where to find what they're seeking.

In the case of Michael's wife, Pearl, the symptoms of AD began with driving aberrations: the car "wasn't holding a steady line" when she drove. Then he began to notice that she became easily disoriented.

> I had to conduct an interview in an office building in downtown Vancouver, and I told Pearl that I shouldn't be more than half an hour so she could wait in the foyer. Well, she went to the washroom there, and the washroom had another exit, which I didn't know about, and when I came to get her, she wasn't there.

> She'd gone. Disappeared . . . She'd gone out through the other
> exit. I forget now how we arranged to locate her, but she was on
> the eighth or tenth floor, going down the stairs. It was a pretty
> scary experience.

Some AD patients are at greater risk of wandering than others. One of the first signs of a potential wanderer is when he/she comes back from a drive or regular walk later than usual. Other strong indicators include talking about going to work at some job the person left long ago, "going home" when he/she is already home or repeatedly asking the whereabouts of current or past friends and family members. You can also expect wandering if the patient paces, is restless or makes repetitive movements, has difficulty locating familiar places like the bathroom, kitchen or bedroom, or becomes nervous or anxious in crowded areas such as shopping malls or restaurants.

You can reduce the possibility of wandering by establishing a regular pattern of exercise and by assigning chores that will keep the patient busy, especially simple things that need to be done regularly like folding laundry and preparing dinner. Make sure all the patient's basic needs—toileting, nutrition and thirst—are met. Never leave a dementia patient unsupervised, try to avoid busy places that can cause disorientation and always provide reassurance as soon as there are signs that he/she feels lost, disoriented or abandoned.

Be sure you control house and car keys because a dementia patient may not wander away only on foot. Place deadbolts on doors either very high or very low because a person with dementia will reach for a lock in the normal waist-high location. Disguise your exterior doors with mirrors or large photographs or even large *No Exit* signs. Consider installing an alarm system triggered by motion or by pressure on the floor mats inside the front and back doors; some caregivers have installed electronically controlled doors and gates. Caregiver Maureen reports that her husband, Merv, has become a "pacer."

> He just paces, paces, paces all night long, up and down. And when
> the weather is good, he is out there walking and walking. Thank
> goodness we live in a large house and it's all fenced and has
> electronic gates so he cannot go out of the grounds because he
> doesn't remember the gate codes anymore.

Finally, if your AD partner is a wanderer, alert the neighbours and ask them to call you if they see your Alzheimer's partner setting off by him/herself.

CHAPTER FOUR

Care Homes

Soon after Clair's first symptoms suggested themselves—mild memory disturbances and the occasional light left on in our apartment—she became fascinated with the idea of labyrinths. When she decided to create one within our garden at Halfmoon Bay, we paced out a tentative design for it together. Then, still connected with this idea, she began subscribing to labyrinth newsletters and magazines. Oblivious to any significance to these events beyond their being the products of her continually active and curious mind, I supported and encouraged her within this fantasy.

The Greeks knew the labyrinth as the structure built by Daedalus to imprison the half-man/half-bull Minotaur, but Daedalus had constructed it so cleverly that for a time he was lost within it himself. Today's labyrinths are composed of a single unambiguous pathway leading to a centre point, and they often represent the possibility of a spiritual journey. I now realize that for Clair the labyrinth may have had allegorical significance as she entered the first chapter of what would be a much longer journey, that she saw it as a spiritual approach through her early befuddlement and confusion. Either consciously or unconsciously—or somewhere in between—her interest in the labyrinth may have represented her courage as she began her search for answers for what was just starting to disturb her.

But the time came when Clair and I could no longer carry on our lives striving for the peaceful centre of her labyrinth. Her AD was worsening and she began following the steps of decompensation—or falling apart—more than once necessitating hospitalization. And after we had lived and loved together for so many wonderful years, she was becoming increasingly irritable, lonely and probably bored after being dissuaded from returning to her high-responsibility job. She began spending Mondays with her sister-in-law Valerie while I worked at the local mental health clinic. The two women were a natural fit, and they almost always seemed to enjoy their time together. Attempts to hire a caregiver for Clair were less successful. Clair decided she was being kidnapped by a caregiver who was in fact driving her home. Plans to invite a cook into our home were shelved after it became clear that Clair was no longer comfortable with strangers in our home. Then she began phoning 911 to report a "stranger" (me) in our house, prompting house calls from the police.

It should have been obvious to me that Clair was no longer comfortable within her own home or within her deteriorating sense of self, and that she was becoming a potential threat to herself or others. Today when I reread my journal from that bleak time in our lives, the significance of events that I missed at the time leaps out at me with striking clarity. But hindsight is always 20/20, isn't it? Neither of us knew it, but she was about eleven months from hospitalization when I penned the first of the following brief notes.

Saturday, January 2, 2010. Clair is labile [unstable] . . . and frustrated with me driving her and [her niece] Nicole home.

Saturday, May 8, 2010. Clair and I read . . . I pour her a whiskey. She has taken off her AD bracelet and discarded it.

Saturday, June 12, 2010. We make love. So close to her. Wow. I bring her fruit salad, muffins and coffee to bed.

Wednesday, August 11, 2010. Clair angry with me re $ [after dinner with friends].

Saturday, September 18, 2010. Some friction with Clair . . . [She is] unhappy with me. [She asks] "Will we marry?" etc. Talk & listen. Lonely. Peace.

Sunday, September 19, 2010. Clair [emotionally] labile. [There are] outburst(s) [but she is] quick to recover.

Saturday, November 27, 2010. We attend the Stuart McLean [performance] with Joy, David and Nicholas. She enjoys [the show but] afterwards at home she explodes. [After a] phone call to [her son] Robert she half-apologizes to me.

Sunday, November 28, 2010. Clair [worries] "What if David comes?" She phones 911 re "a stranger in our house!" [This is her fifth call to the RCMP or West Vancouver Police Department in the past six to eight weeks.] The RCMP constable urges her to see her MD tomorrow. [Afterwards] I am David again.

Monday, November 29, 2010. Good [clinic] day . . . Pick up Clair at Valerie's. Then to ferry at Langdale, to Horseshoe Bay and to Lions Gate Hospital [in North Vancouver]. Psych rounds in less than 6 hours. Peace. Amen.

Tuesday, November 30, 2010. The new attending MD in ER transfers Clair to 2-W. She is agitated, irritable, up and down.

Wednesday, December 1, 2010. I visit a rested Clair.

Thursday, December 2, 2010. Took clothes to Clair [but] forgot some. She is angry, defiant [with all of us]. [Another] 911 outburst.

Clair would not be coming home again. Within three months—a period that included an attempt to escape from Lions Gate Hospital associated with an aggressive encounter with hospital security—she was transferred to a private room at the Kiwanis Care Centre (KCC), midway between North Vancouver and Deep Cove on Burrard Inlet. Clair's family, including me, were extremely pleased at finding a bed for her in Cypress Cove, a secure "nursing neighbourhood" within KCC. It was our first choice, and the staff displayed a super blend of warmth and professionalism.

In a dementia unit, ward or neighbourhood there are often individuals in distress, agitated, lonely, crying out or trying to articulate some inner lost, lonely or confused part of their private experience. And Clair, who in her early days there had not lost her warm and empathetic mental health instincts, would often approach one of these individuals, trying to comfort them, massaging an arm tenderly or perhaps mumbling a few kind words. Not all residents would respond appreciatively to her gestures, though, and would occasionally push back. At which point Clair would deck them, frequently knocking their unappreciative selves to the floor. Soon enough I would receive a phone call from the charge nurse, informing me that "David, Clair has been . . . uh. . . aggressive." I would hang up the phone after this news with only one thought: *she's still Clair!*

Could we have waited longer before placing her in care? How much longer? And at what price for her family, for me and most of all for Clair herself? In the caregivers' support group to which I belong, there are three groups. The members of the first are committed to keeping their loved ones at home, come what may. Many of them have daytime care assistance or a twenty-four-hour live-in care aide who works maybe eight to ten hours a day but is also available for unofficial backup should an urgent need arise. The second group's members might have started in a position similar to those in the first group, but opted for placement after realizing the enormous and increasing difficulties involved in keeping their AD loved ones at home. The third group's members hover halfway between group one and group two. They find themselves increasingly conflicted about placement as their partners present new challenges and difficulties each month, if not each day. And they themselves often experience increasing mental, emotional and physical problems associated with the stress, strain and conflict they are experiencing.

Graham's wife had died about thirteen months before I interviewed him for this book. As he had been a member of a support organization to which I belonged, I already knew he was one of the caregivers in that first group, those committed to caring for their partners at home. When I commented on how sharply he had been focused on this, he said,

> I don't think I made Yvonne any promises that I would keep
> her at home, and certainly even if I had, I would probably have
> broken them if that had been necessary to keep me alive. But I
> preferred to keep her at home, and quite frankly I believe that
> it's easier at home. That is, for me. I'm not saying it would be for
> everybody, but for me it was probably easier at home because
> I'm something of a control freak as a personality type, and when
> she was at home, I could run the show. I could determine what we
> were going to do with Yvonne and what we weren't going to do.
> That includes medication, it includes how she was treated, what
> she wore and what she did every day . . . that kind of stuff. I never
> consciously listed all the reasons why I wanted to keep her at
> home, but I just wanted to do that, and as the disease progressed,
> I continued to feel that way. My brother said the other day—and
> he is absolutely correct—that I took a great deal of pride in being
> able to keep her at home the whole time because I knew she'd be
> happier here. And she was. Even though lots of people thought I
> was crazy, and it was really, really hard on me, I didn't find it nearly
> as difficult as I think I would have found putting her into a facility.

Commenting on his more recent role as support and mentor for other men/caregivers of AD partners, Graham says,

> I would very much like to encourage people—not all people, but
> those who are able—to keep their spouses at home. I think it's a

much healthier place . . . and I think it's a much more rewarding thing if you can do it. But as I say, not all people can, but the younger ones can. The two guys I'm working with—one's sixty-six and the other's sixty-two—they're managing at home quite well. And for both of them I'm probably the cause of why they're doing it because I was able to show them how to do it.

Of course, not everyone is equipped by temperament for a caregiving role, or in a financial position to stay home as a caregiver. My friend Graham, in spite of being sure that keeping his own wife at home was the correct choice in his case, was not adamant that everyone should do what he did. He told me,

There was one guy in our men's group who kept his wife at home for a long time and then he finally gave up and put her in a facility. And he came to me privately after he did that—about six or eight months after that—and he said, "I just want to say thank you." And I said, "What do you mean?" And he said, "Well, you gave me the strength and the commitment to be able to put my wife in a home. Even though you didn't do it yourself, you encouraged me to do it for a number of reasons. And I want to thank you because you saved my life and improved my relationship with my wife."

Many of the other caregivers I interviewed for this book were likely in the third category, conflicted about whether to place their partners in care, anxious about the quality of care available in a facility, worried that the personnel in a care home would not understand the limitations or unmanageable behaviour of their loved ones. John, whose wife was diagnosed with AD eight years ago, told me,

Well, I guess I've always said in my heart I want to keep her at home to the very end, but I'm not sure I'm strong enough for that. What I saw a friend go through . . . I'm not sure I could go that far with her if she goes down as far as his wife did. On the other hand, I'm not convinced that most of the care homes would look after her the way I'm caring for her. I'm worried about over-medication, I'm worried about how she would react to rigid rules and routines. She won't get the love or the coddling that she gets at home. Like when she's eating if she's . . . You know, [at home] there's no definite timeframe with meals. She can spend as long as she likes. She usually eats pretty well, but occasionally all she wants to do is mix the food up on the plate, and it doesn't get up to her mouth, you know?

With mostly hindsight, I appreciate now that I, like John, had been a member of that third group for some time before I drove Clair to the hospital in November 2010. In retrospect, I can see how easy it was to overlook the big picture of her needs in my own loneliness, depression and anticipatory grief. In the end, it was only the process of more sharply weighing my needs against hers that allowed me to move from the third group to the second group. The big questions that most caregivers fail to ask before they get to that point are these:

- What are my loved one's needs for continuity of care, kindness and help?
- How much does she/he seem to be enjoying time at home?
- What does she/he deserve?
- What price am I paying in my own health and well-being?
- How much am *I* enjoying this experience at home?

These questions are often preempted by denial, a longing for earlier times or an unwillingness or inability to balance our partner's needs with our own. When our own mental or medical health takes a serious regression, or it finally becomes apparent that our partner's needs can no longer be adequately met at home, it is time to take a few steps:

- a consultation with the family doctor and, if possible, with a geriatrician, gerontologist or geriatric psychiatrist;
- meetings with family and close friends;
- meditation or prayer, if it is appropriate for you;
- talking more openly with whatever caregiver support group you belong to;
- visits to a counsellor or therapist for help in understanding the mixed feelings or conflicts surrounding all of the above (rather than sweeping them under the carpet);
- visits to at least a few caregiving homes, talking to staff there and, if possible, also with family members whose own loved ones are now living comfortably in placement (and listening to those family members' accounts of their own placement conflicts and experiences, both positive and negative).

Last, but far from least, with the above help and support, and also on your own, examine the many ways in which placement may be not only to your advantage but to your partner's advantage. A win–win situation.

Now go ahead and say that word out loud once or twice. Placement. **Placement**. That wasn't too bad, was it? It can be a tough slog for those of you who have yet to face this big decision, yet it doesn't have to be weighty.

In the end, it wasn't weighty for me. Although experiencing sadness, loss and loneliness, grief and regret, I also felt enormous relief when I took Clair to the Lions Gate Hospital emergency department that night—relief that she would not call 911 again from our home (although she would try it from the hospital once or twice), and probably some relief that she would no longer experience terror about the stranger (me) living in our home, a terror that was forcing her to phone the police.

Some of my friends' AD partners continue to live at home with them, sometimes with enormous associated stress on one or both of them, and I find myself a little more critical now that I can see the forest for the trees in my own case, now that I don't have to help Clair get toileted and dressed or undressed for bed. I reminded my caregiver support group last week— stopping short of lecturing, though, I hope—that there are only five questions about placement (a word rarely used in our group) facing those of us whose partners continue to live at home. First, *is this what you want?* Second, *do you think this is also what your partner wants—and needs?* Third, *are you up to keeping your partner at home?* Can you do this day in and day out, perhaps with the help of your live-in care aide, for years and years? Fourth, *have you asked your care aide what her/his feelings are about your decision and discussed it with her/him in any detail?* And fifth and finally, *at what price will you continue to keep your partner at home?* What is that price for your partner, your care aide and not least yourself?

Of course, these same questions need to be faced about the opposite option—placing your partner in a home. For me it was more or less a straightforward set of questions and answers; keeping Clair at home would have been unkind not only to her but to me. For those of you standing at this crossroads, things might not appear so clear. You can see that your partner still needs you physically and perhaps emotionally as well. But how much do you need him or her physically? Probably less and less as the dementia worsens in the progressive manner typical and predictable for AD. And how much do you need her/him emotionally? A small amount? Maybe a moderate amount or a lot? Of course, you don't have to be emotionally dependent to want your partner to stay at home with you. It may be a matter of love, neediness, familiarity with family and marriage traditions and a certain overt or covert need for that to continue. And it's okay to consciously need your partner to be at home with you, too—to a degree. But the key word here is *consciously*. If you are mostly aware of your own mental and emotional wiring, then you are in a good, strong position to be able to wrestle with the questions listed above.

So how do you gauge that all-important level of awareness of your inner feelings, needs, conflicts and emotional makeup? Listen to your dreams. Listen to those family members or friends you trust and respect the most.

If your placement decision doesn't work out, if the placement pieces or timetables don't seem to fall comfortably together, or if some trusted friends or family members have strong feelings about your placement decisions (or about the comfort—or lack of it—that often comes with having made a choice), then consulting a counsellor can help bring you wisdom and insight about both your external and internal self and dynamics. And if you have joined a caregivers' support group—I strongly recommend joining one—you can benefit from the experiences, conflicts, thoughts and emotions that others have faced in the recent or distant past, are currently struggling with or may be anticipating confronting in the near or intermediate future.

Don't forget to share your own experiences and conflicts. I have found that whether I'm attending formal or informal get-togethers, coffee sessions or meetings with others facing this dilemma, what they have to say is most helpful when I keep my ears open, listen sharply and try not to give advice. At such times removing my doctor's hat is most useful, and I seem to learn more when I'm talking less and listening more closely to other people's experiences and situations.

So how are you feeling about all this right now? How are you thinking? Are you relaxed, comfortable and (mostly) anxiety free (or at least at a low anxiety point on your scale)? Do you and your beloved need each other about the same as you did, say, ten years ago? Not much more but not much less? Are you as comfortable with him or her as you were, say, a year ago? Is there still a palpable warmth between you? Do you still have certain ways in which you seem to connect with each other? Are you rested, content and happy? Are you experiencing not many more physical or emotional symptoms than those you reported to your family doctor, say, six to eight years ago? Not wrestling with more guilt feelings than is usual for you? Are you seeing a counsellor when you want to or need to? Are you keeping up to date with your chums, friends and important peer groups?

If the answers to the above questions are mostly positive, then you have probably made—or are probably making—the right placement decisions.

|||||||||||||||||||||||||||||||

No one challenged Clair's family and me in our thinking about her placement. Her doctors supported us. Our community and family were there for us. And when after twelve weeks she was transferred from the hospital to the Kiwanis Care Centre, she and I went down on our knees next to her new bed to offer prayers of gratitude. And we made love, one of the last times we would share that intimacy. It was then that the quiet thought I had pushed to the back of my mind was finally confirmed: she and I would not be together at home again. Ever. But the decisions, important checkpoints, discussions and problem-solving with Clair, her family, my family and step-family, and our separate and overlapping sets of friends had all preceded that final decision concerning where she would live for the rest of her life. With hindsight, it is clear to me that the decisions we all had to—or were privileged to—make had fallen into one or more of eight separate categories of pondering and reflection.

These are the eight most important ways to approach, or even think about, placement. First and second, what are the pluses and the minuses around your partner going into a care home or facility soon? Third and fourth, what are the pros and the cons regarding your partner *not* going into a facility, but staying at home for now? Fifth and sixth, what are the pluses and the minuses for *your* mental, emotional and physical well-being should your partner go into care? Seventh and eighth, what are the pros and the cons for *your* well-being should your partner remain at home?

Let us remember—and forgive me for possibly restating the obvious— that your partner will likely have difficulty verbalizing any thoughts or reactions to the questions I've just listed. At the same time, your own consideration of these questions may be clouded by your neediness, anxiety, projections, loneliness and more. Perhaps you want to put your partner in a home today without delay. Are you possibly being a little impatient in this decision? For what reasons? Or perhaps you say you will never put your partner in a home. Is this for his/her benefit, or is it related to underlying emotional, altruistic or dependency conflicts that you may not be fully in touch with?

Think it through carefully. Perhaps write down the pros and cons. Other than your decision to become partners in the first place, this is the most important decision in all your years together, so take all the time you need.

||||||||||||||||||||||||||||||||

So how does one find a care home? Start your search *early* among the members of your caregiver support group, where experience abounds. Talk with your family physician, who has probably been through this conversation many, many times with other patients and their families. Visit several homes—if possible in your part of town. Talk to the staff and, if you're allowed, to the residents as well. Should you bring your partner with you? That will have to be your judgement call. But whatever you do, listen to your intuition, your experience and your insight. And honour all of them.

The cost of residences can vary widely. Clair lives in a residence overseen by the Vancouver Coastal Health Authority. Although it is a public agency, families are expected to pay on a sliding scale, but the cost is still about one-third to one-half of what we would be paying in one of Vancouver's private care residences. Because Clair was still aggressive and at times a wanderer when she was placed, she was admitted to a secure care unit. Other units or nursing neighbourhoods within KCC offer a variety of security arrangements. But it is important to inquire about the versatility and flexibility of units within the residence when you are window-shopping for the most versatile, appropriate residence for your loved one.

The physical plant of the care facility is very important. Is the residence you are considering for your partner clean? Is it well looked after, with a comfortable temperature? And what about the outside places, the gardens and patios where your loved one may be allowed to walk and visit safely? How are the meals? Try one or two yourself, perhaps together with your partner. Do the other residents seem happy? Alert? Lively? The unit where your partner might live for the rest of his/her life will have an indefinable *something* that words cannot always describe, but you or your partner will almost certainly know and appreciate a positive milieu when you see and experience it. Will your partner have a single room of her/his own, as Clair does, or will she/he be expected to share a space with another resident? These are questions that are not always answered quickly or easily, but they *must* be asked, and the earlier in your shared experience that you do this, the better.

Finally, although it is very important to check out the premises, surroundings and physical plant, you should focus on the factor that makes the real difference in a care residence: the staff. Certain nurses, nursing aides, social workers, cooks, recreational and musical therapists and physiotherapists seem to be able to exist comfortably and effectively within care residences for individuals wrestling with (often) progressive dementia. For these people, working with those wounded by dementia is a privilege, and they are the ones you want to have working with your loved one day in and day out. They have a warm respect for people with dementia that is almost always evident when you spend time with them. When listening to your partner, they might paraphrase what they are hearing, but they never rephrase it. They do not scold, criticize or lecture the individuals within their sphere of care; they often share their sense of humour, and as much as is possible they are alert to possibilities of mutuality with their clients.

For some health care workers, all of these attributes seem to be natural, almost intuitive, and they are quite comfortable in their daily work. Other workers may take a little time to adjust completely to the ups and downs of working with dementia patients, but the ones who are destined for this calling are generally fast learners and usually arrive quickly at the acme of dementia care: they soon enjoy their work and are happy sharing with colleagues and with those whose care is entrusted to them. What I have experienced and thoroughly enjoyed watching at KCC is the outstanding leaders and staff and the way they combine warmth and professionalism in such a caring and thoughtful manner. Both your partner and you deserve this much as well.

Other staff who have made a difference to Clair include a music therapist and her assistant because music is such an important way to connect with those with AD. People with Alzheimer's appreciate—and seem to recognize—musical contact and communication in a way that increases its importance as verbal skills decline. (Recently I was invited to join the gang in Clair's unit dancing—what fun!) KCC also provides the services of a social worker, a podiatrist, a manicurist and a hairdresser who visit on a regular basis. A volunteer companion also visits, spending one-on-one time that both she and Clair seem to enjoy. In addition, I arranged for both a gifted massage therapist and a yoga therapist to visit Clair every two weeks. To my regret, when staff became aware that Clair was increasingly uncomfortable with physical contact, the massage visits were cancelled.

You should also get to know your partner's physicians, who have the final responsibility for her/his care. Do they visit regularly? Do they keep in touch with the charge nurse? What is their philosophy regarding psychotropic medications? Do they routinely sedate their patients prophylactically, or do they strive for a dynamic balance, helping their patients to live in the residence with as little sedation as possible, prescribing only on an as-needed (*pro re nata* or PRN) basis when the patient becomes aggressive? Do they review medications regularly, including sedatives and psychotropic medication, using feedback from the staff combined with their own observations, experience and intuition?

All of these factors are important for the well-being of your loved one, but you should also have periodic family meetings with the staff. They are in touch with your partner's treating physicians on a regular basis and help keep her/his care up to date, fresh and appropriate. They also have the deepest shared respect for your partner.

CHAPTER FIVE

Improving Your AD Partner's Quality of Life

When at times two become one,
I am reminded that the F-word is Fun.

It's Tuesday evening, February 28, 2012. Clair and I have a special engagement this evening, a reservation at the Burr Place Bistro. This is "an opportunity for residents and their guests to enjoy a fine dining experience without leaving KCC. The Kiwanis Room is transformed into an elegant dining room, a chef prepares a delicious three-course meal and wine is complementary."

We sneak in a gourmet appetizer—a twenty-minute snuggle in her room. I do most of the kissing, but that's fine by me. And I try some light petting without a strong positive response from Clair. So—off to the Burr Place Bistro we go!

> CLAIR: "Are we going out tonight?"
>
> ME: "Yes, and we're also going in. It's a dining date for us, my love! You are my date!"

Clair and I are both intrigued by the elegant menu, a copy of which each of us kept.

Burr Place Bistro
February 28, 2012
Bocconcini Tomato Skewers
With Basil, Olive Oil and Balsamic Vinegar
Salmon with Mushrooms and
Spinach Wrapped in Puff Pastry
Served with Asparagus and Rice Pilaf
OR
Pork Chops and Apples in a Sage Cream Sauce
Served with Maple Glazed Carrots and Roasted Red Potatoes

⌒✳︎⌒

Chocolate Lava Cakes
With Whipped Cream

Clair struggles with her menu choice but eventually chooses the pork. Both of us opt for a glass of red wine to go with our meal. While waiting between courses, I ask her to dance. She wriggles out of her chair, and we waltz slowly, closely and warmly to the marvellous Platters hit "The Great Pretender." As she lets me gently spin her around the dining room, she twirls gracefully. We sit down after four or five minutes to a round of appreciative applause from our dinner mates. Clair then picks slowly through her food while I enjoy my salmon entrée. But even more than that, I am enjoying the time out with my love. We are on a date, by golly!

As if reading my thoughts, she hesitantly shares, "I'd . . . like to have . . . lunch with you . . . sometime."

"Count me in, dear!" I answer quickly from my heart. Something about getting out of her nursing neighbourhood, however briefly, seems to have loosened both of us up and helped bring us closer together.

She also offers spontaneously a thought about her late beloved brother: "Hugh . . . always wanted . . . his kids nearby!"

I listen and reflect.

And then she says, "Are you tired?"

"Not tired of you. I love you!" I answer freely. Again I feel closer to her, out on our own here. The wonderful nurses provide the warmest, most professional environment for her and the other patients in her nursing neighbourhood, but this evening is different, and we both are enjoying the moment.

"I had a call about . . . an Oak . . . Street event . . . tomorrow, I think," she offers quietly—in regard to I don't know what. And then, "Robert went away . . . and here . . ." (She points at her chocolate lava dessert cake.)

"Uhmm-hmm!" I offer, not knowing how else to respond, though wanting to keep in touch with her, but her voice is diminishing and she is mute for much of the rest of our dinner. She drinks little of her wine but takes four to five sips of her coffee with cream and sugar before we head back to her home quarters in Cypress Cove. I guide her to a seat within occupational therapist Peter's current-events discussion group, and then I slip into her room to place her name card from tonight's memorable dinner on top of her chest of drawers.

I nod to her on the way out, then turn back to kiss her on the top of her head from behind before letting myself out. Walking to the bus stop, I feel refreshed, even upbeat. Now that was a *real date!* I tell myself. But more importantly, I am hoping that this evening made a difference to Clair, too. There is still much I can do to provide companionship, comfort, open communication and, while we're at it, fun for Clair.

|||||||||||||||||||||||||||||||

You can find the same kind of opportunities for your AD partner within your community as well—even after he/she is in a care facility. And while it may seem like an oxymoron to have fun with a partner suffering from dementia, believe me, it's a wonderful way to take care of yourself at the same time as improving your partner's quality of life. In this chapter I want to share some of the ways I've learned to have fun with Clair since her diagnosis and, more importantly, since she entered the care facility.

Reading

Clair and I have always loved to read, though maybe she enjoyed it more than I did (and do), especially Alice Munro's short stories. But as her AD progressed, she lost most of the initiative, appreciation and proactivity that in the past would see her eagerly buy, rent and borrow books or share them with the people she loved. On a few occasions after she first entered KCC, I would see her scanning a section of the *Vancouver Sun* newspaper. Then no more. For a few months after that I tried reading to her but gave up, unsure whether we were connecting. Later I wondered if maybe, just maybe, I had been over-reading—or under-reading—her body messages, if maybe I had been somewhat insensitive to the nonverbal messages that our snuggling tutorials since then have helped me with. And recently I learned of studies that showed how reading to those with Alzheimer's disease can increase their ability to engage with others.

Some studies suggest it may be enough to read to your partner from a favourite book, but now there are also books available that have been specifically designed to be read to dementia sufferers. *The Sunshine on My Face: A Read-Aloud Book for Memory-Challenged Adults* was written by Lydia Burdick, who wanted something to read to her own mother when she was in the late stages of Alzheimer's disease. Burdick had discovered that when well-meaning caregivers and hospital staff read children's books to dementia patients, most of these patients turned away, having found the experience "insulting and demeaning" because the books didn't reflect the life experiences of adults. Although her own book has large print and colourful illustrations, it features adults participating in adult activities. Another good book is *A Little, Aloud: An Anthology of Prose and Poetry for Reading Aloud to Someone You Care For* (Chatto & Windus, 2010). The excerpts in this one range from Shakespeare to *Black Beauty*, each one chosen by editor Angela MacMillan to appeal to dementia patients.

Learning more about the value of reading to Alzheimer's patients prompted me to take some short stories by Alice Munro out to KCC the next night when I went to visit Clair. Later I tried reading a portion of *The Sunshine on My Face*, which as Clair's disease progressed seemed more appropriate. And she smiled widely when quite recently I read her my eleven-year-old poem "My Clair." And I certainly enjoyed reading it to her for probably the first time in ten years. It had been my poetic response after she had half-apologized one long-ago March afternoon for "not being a nicer person." I wrote:

> *You know something? IF I had wanted nice, I'd have asked*
> > *for:*
> *• Mary Poppins, or*
> *• the Tooth Fairy, or*
> *• Somebody Else.*
> *Instead—I married:*
> *• Amelia Earhart and*
> *• Martha Stewart and*
> *• Clair Huxtable*
> *• Golda Meier*
> *• Kim Campbell*
> *• Rosa Parks, and*
> *• Pauline Johnson*
> *• Isabel Gunn and*
> *• Sacagawea and*
> *• Annie Oakley, and . . .*
> *More. So much, so many more.*
> *You know something?*
> *I'm a lucky guy.*
>
> *David, March 29, 2002*

Music and Dancing

More than reading to Clair, however, for a long time after she moved to KCC I felt comfortable connecting with her through music. She never seemed to tire of my singing Irving Berlin's "(I Wonder Why) You're Just in Love." Or maybe I never got tired of warbling it to her? Probably both. And I remember singing Don Robertson's "Hummingbird" to her, changing a few possibly hurtful words along the way. What is just as interesting and helps remind us that music reaches out to both caregiver and AD partner is that I also found myself singing Peter, Paul and Mary's version of "The Fox" to her, to myself and sometimes to anyone who would listen while I was on my way to the bus stop.

Dancing with Clair during her first years at KCC was always a treat. With our first velvety move around Crescent Cove's floor, she would snuggle easily into my arms and dance with me to the sounds of our wonderful musical therapists on their electric keyboards. I felt so connected to her as we waltzed happily across the floor, and she seemed to appreciate my singing sweet nothings softly into her ear while we danced. Recent research would seem to agree with what Clair and I discovered on our own: that, especially for people with AD struggling with anxiety or depression, music and dancing are great medicine.

The Alzheimer's Foundation of America website explains that engaging Alzheimer's patients in music activities can spark compelling outcomes even in the very late stages of the disease because music doesn't require "cognitive or mental processing." In fact, according the website, music, and particularly rhythm playing and singing, "can shift mood, manage stress-induced agitation, stimulate positive interactions, facilitate cognitive function, and coordinate motor movements . . . As dementia progresses, individuals typically lose the ability to share thoughts and gestures of affection with their loved ones. However, they retain their ability to move with the beat until very late in the disease process."

One study has shown that dementia and Alzheimer's patients can recall memories and emotions and demonstrate enhanced mental performance after singing tunes from old movies and musicals.[1] In this study the researchers led half of the patients through selected songs while the other half just listened. Afterwards, all of them took cognitive ability and life satisfaction tests, which showed that those who sang did "significantly better" than those who just listened. The researchers also discovered that the show tunes that had the greatest effect were those patients had enjoyed most before they developed dementia. It was another sign that, as therapy, singing is cheap, effortless and very productive.

Physical Contact

Therapists stress the importance of warm, positive physical contact between you and your loved one for as long as you both are comfortable with it. For several years when visiting Clair, I would quickly invite her to join me on her bed, and she usually agreed. Later I became more judicious and would spell out my invitations more slowly and carefully, reminding her that, like me, she had choices. Learning from Clair's nonverbal snuggling or cuddling messages soon taught me to be more circumspect with her. For example, after a time she didn't seem to spoon with me as warmly and naturally as she once did, sometimes firmly separating the lower half of her body from mine. In addition, after she allowed me to remove her shoes before we hopped into bed, she would often replace them before slipping back into bed and snuggling with me. Mostly we laughed about this together, which probably helped to reduce the tension and any discomfort that either of us was experiencing.

Rich O'Boyle of Elder Care Online notes that touching one's Alzheimer's partner need not be reserved for expressing sexual interest. Touching can also convey such things as compassion, safety and reassurance as well as providing a signal to relax. He reminds caregivers always to maintain physical contact—holding a hand or arm—with their loved ones when standing or sitting with them. He also suggests massaging scented lotion into the patient's hands and especially the feet because old people's feet don't often get touched.

Before her placement, Clair and I had studied yoga with a teacher we both liked and respected; today that teacher continues to visit Clair every other week and then reports back to me with a summary of their latest session. I don't understand all that they do together, but I respect their work and have a sense that this therapist is connecting with Clair in a way that perhaps no one else is now able to.

What about finding a part-time companion for your AD partner? Clair's companion, who visits her one on one twice weekly, is one of the many professionals who work at KCC. I think these companions are chosen for this job because they are warm, quiet and comfortable people who have a special wavelength with the patients there. What does she do with Clair? Almost anything two friends would do. Hang out. Go for walks. Accompany her on field trips and outings. In addition, after Clair began to have difficulty feeding herself, her companion attended more regularly to help feed her.

Visits from Family Pets

Most care homes are happy to have visits from well-behaved (and leashed!) family pets, especially dogs, because such visits almost always elicit a positive response. Margaret and her husband, Donald, had always walked their two dogs together before he was placed in care. She told me,

> Donald didn't really like to muck around in the barn [with the horses] or do any of that, but we always walked the dogs together until he couldn't any more. He loved his dogs. [After he was in care] I would take them down to the care home because he loved to visit with them and talk to them and pet them . . . It doesn't matter what mood you're in, if you're sad, if you're happy, if you're tired, [dogs] are there, wagging their tails.

Therapy Animals

A growing number of hospitals and care homes are accepting visits from well-trained dogs, and sometimes cats, because of their calming effect on patients, particularly those with Alzheimer's or other forms of dementia. Petting and stroking a soft, furry animal is known to slow the heart rate, lower blood pressure, reduce the stress hormone cortisol and boost levels of the feel-good hormone serotonin.

Researchers from the College of Nursing at the University of Nebraska Medical Center discovered that dogs could help Alzheimer's patients experiencing sundown syndrome.[2] Sundown syndrome is characterized by aimless wandering, confusion, agitation and aggressive behaviour such as hitting, kicking and biting; it affects some Alzheimer's patients in early evening. Such behaviour often leads to social isolation, which may in turn lead to more aggressiveness. Doctors have traditionally administered drugs to deal with this condition, but the UNMC researchers, focusing on twenty-eight patients in three extended-care facilities, showed that a therapy dog could produce the same results, reducing stress and providing affection and companionship. The researchers suggested that home caregivers might also want to consider acquiring a therapy dog because home patients often suffer from isolation and loneliness.

Laughter

Humour is good not only for your AD partner but for you as well. Just remember that the things you find funny, your partner with AD may no longer find funny. I also had to learn that just because Clair was laughing, it didn't mean I had to laugh, and just because she was not laughing, it didn't mean I couldn't laugh out loud, guffaw and enjoy the moment. This was all great practice in reminding myself where Clair stopped and I started. And where I started and she stopped.

For a long time Clair and I would have fun flirting, teasing and laughing with each other. I enjoyed teasing her, tickling her, uttering raunchy yet sincere and heartfelt sweet nothings in her ear (this would never fail to get a reaction!) and just talking to her and with her on a lighter note. I felt closer to her when one or both of us were laughing or giggling, and I shared that feeling of closeness with her. Humour is certainly a language she not only understood but enjoyed. In this way, she was still Clair. One day when she and our friend Joy were dancing, Joy stepped on her toes. Clair commented, "I was wondering how long it would be before you did that!" This was followed by guffaws, giggles and hugs by both!

Laughing *with* someone who is struggling with such a cruel disease? Why not? The long-term prognosis is bad, even sad and scary, but that should not keep us from the gift of living in the moment with our loved ones. I came to realize and appreciate that the moment, the here and now, was all that Clair and I could still share with each other. So why not enjoy it? A lot.

As I was writing these words, a Zen koan came to mind, sort of a parable about life and living in the moment, and it goes something like this:

> A man travelling across a field encountered a tiger. He fled, the tiger after him. Coming to a precipice, he caught hold of the root of a wild vine and swung himself down over the edge. The tiger sniffed at him from above. Trembling, the man looked down to where, far below, another tiger was waiting to eat him. Only the vine sustained him. But two mice started to gnaw away the vine. Just then the man saw a luscious strawberry near him. Grasping the vine with one hand, he plucked the strawberry with the other. How sweet it tasted!

Finally, overlapping with many if not all of the above suggestions for improving your AD partner's life in care is the life-giving gift of intimacy and closeness. Does this seem remote, like something you've already given up on? I know I had begun to give up on the possibility of closeness with Clair after her first year or so in care. Then I experienced the most wonderful sensations in singing or dancing or just being silly with her. Just being with her. It seems as though I was still growing, letting myself be a better David, a better husband, a better partner and a better friend.

CHAPTER SIX

Taking Care of the Caregiver

A toast:

Here's to Aloneness
and her second cousin, Loneliness.
May we continue to especially savour and enjoy the former
Without being absorbed by the latter.

After Clair was first diagnosed with Alzheimer's disease, many friends and family members reminded or cautioned me, "David, be sure and take care of yourself!" But how does that—how did that—translate into behavioural changes, into actual operations and procedures in my life? How do we as caregivers transform "taking care of ourselves" into a program that is not only meaningful but also helpful, supportive and perhaps even comforting?

At that time I was working harder than ever in two separate mental health offices. In the evening I was busy charting notes, buying groceries, keeping in touch with my children in Oregon and with friends and other family in Vancouver and elsewhere. But I missed Clair on so many levels, and as she continued to disappear, I ached, hungered for her and our old days. When I visited her, we still snuggled and I would sing to her. Yet at the same time I was losing her, so my centre, my focus, my person and—on some days—my journal all paid the price. The words were there, but the sentences were threadbare. If the sentences were there, the overview of the day itself was sparse. And when those days were wonderfully there, there was no guarantee that tomorrow would start or end with a similar, meaningful, warm or important focus. As a result, my journal became less important. What was the point of writing it by myself without Clair next to me in bed to bounce off ideas, to laugh with as we shared and reviewed our often close and overlapping days?

Behind this vacuum was the backstory of the emptiness in my life, which I appreciated only poorly then. With Clair gone, I failed to realize that I—me, myself—was still a real, honest-to-goodness human being with feelings, conflicts, hopes and needs. Intellectually, somewhere in my left brain, I knew this and appreciated it, but the rest of me—the emotional, physical, spiritual, sexual and social parts of me—had been lost in the shuffle, had become numb.

My problems in taking care of myself, however, did not manifest themselves until well after Clair was admitted to North Vancouver's Lions Gate Hospital. Rather than experience or deal with conflict while Clair's destiny was in transition, I seem to have waited to become symptomatic until after many of my tears were shed and my teeth were mostly finished gnashing. I had pushed my conflicts about her care and eventual placement out of my conscious mind, stuffing those feelings down deep and keeping them there by overworking to the point of exhaustion. Then, less than six weeks after she moved into care, I began walking in my sleep, something completely new to me. The sleepwalking would turn out to correlate with a previously undiagnosed complex fatigue syndrome.

After I started sleepwalking, I conducted one or two bad psychotherapy sessions, but I still had zero insight into how I was—or wasn't—doing. Then one day a patient and I were reviewing her previous, disturbing session during which I had not been fully present, yet I had actually written down her concerns in my chart notes: "David, is something the matter?" she had said. "David, should we cancel this session?" Though I had written her words down, I had absolutely no memory of these events.

I took some time off after that to think about my situation. In the first week of October 2011, my son Andy came from Oregon to visit me, and over Sunday breakfast he and our friend Jay announced they were taking me to Vancouver General Hospital. "Okay," I said. Then I shrugged. I had no idea why they were so concerned about me because I was totally unaware of the absent, drooling spell they had been witnessing. What followed were eleven days of multi-specialty workups, spinal taps, head scans of various types and consultations with psychiatrists, neurologists, geriatricians and more. I was discharged with diagnoses of multiple neurological disorders including temporal lobe epilepsy combined with central sleep apnea, in which my brain was forgetting to tell my chest muscles to breathe.

The follow-up was challenging and demanding but rewarding. And with positive results away went my borderline delusion that caregiver fatigue and exhaustion are things that happen to somebody else. Even more importantly, that eleven-day hospital experience served to remind me what I had conveniently and semi-comfortably forgotten: that I, like every human being, have emotional, spiritual and physical strengths, but also vulnerabilities.

That hospitalization was followed by an eleven-month sick leave, time off that proved to be one large blessing or a series of small blessings in disguise. I decelerated. I sold my car and began visiting Clair by bus. Once I overcame my initial frustrations with bus schedules and connections and enduring sometimes-cold temperatures while I waited at bus stops, I began to enjoy riding with other passengers, experiencing the wide variety of humanity close up, from angels to assholes. I gained a lot of respect for the drivers. I enjoyed watching moms and nannies climbing on board with their charges in prams, and older folks easing their way into the bus with their walkers and packages. I talked to other riders on the bus, noticing the beauty of children and their caregivers, something I'd neither seen nor focused on as I whizzed through life on autopilot at eighty kilometres an hour with—and then without—Clair.

|||||||||||||||||||||||||||||||||||

In the Alzheimer's game, the stakes are, or can be, very high for care-givers. A substantial body of research shows that family members who provide care to individuals with chronic or disabling conditions are them-selves at high risk of illness. Depending on the methodology of the study, researchers have placed the number of caregivers—usually spouses—who will die before their AD partners at somewhere between 30 and 50 percent. A study by the AARP Public Policy Institute gives caregivers a death rate 63 percent higher than non-caregivers in the same age group.[1] Caregivers who experience chronic stress may be at greater risk for cognitive decline themselves, including losses in short-term memory, attention span and verbal IQ. There are also special cardiovascular risks that caregivers—espe-cially women—face, but caregivers of both sexes exhibit exaggerated car-diovascular responses to stressful conditions, which puts them at greater risk than non-caregivers for the development of cardiovascular syndromes such as high blood pressure or heart disease. In fact, women who spend nine or more hours a week caring for an ill or disabled spouse increase their risk of heart disease twofold. In a 2011 US study, between 17 and 35 percent of caregivers reported their health as fair or poor, with one or more chronic conditions or a disability and chronic conditions (including heart attack/heart disease, cancer, diabetes and arthritis) at nearly twice the rate of non-caregivers.[2]

For Maureen, the pros and cons of placing her husband, Merv, in a care home weighed heavily on her because of her own poor health.

> What worries me the most is not being able to take care of him properly myself and not being able to cope as I'd like to, not to lose my patience—and that's pretty hard for me sometimes. Because I'm not that well, and he's, you know, boom, boom, boom! Every five minutes he's losing everything. It's a bombardment all day whether the [hired] caregiver is there or not. I need to take care of him and sometimes I resent that. When I speak to him and he becomes confrontational, he will call me every name in the book—and then he doesn't remember any of it. I try not to activate the confrontations. I just try to go along and reassure him all the time that everything's fine, but he'll wake up in the night yelling as if something terrible is happening, and I quiet him down . . . that's all I can do . . . I believe he will outlive me by many years. I have heart problems and I'm not able to breathe too well. I was going to the gym, but I had knee surgery again . . . So probably the best thing would be for me to put him in a home and try to heal myself for a while. I am trying to put everything in perspective, but I guess I would always feel guilty about [placing him in care].

Caregivers suffer from an increased rate of physical ailments (including acid reflux, headaches and other pain), an increased tendency to develop serious illness and higher levels of obesity. Studies also demonstrate that caregivers have a diminished immune response and slower wound healing, which lead to frequent and longer infections and increased risk of cancers. They also have a higher level of stress hormones and a lower level of antibody responses. On top of this, the physical strain of caregiving can also have an effect, especially when the caregiver is providing care for someone who cannot transfer him/herself out of bed, walk or bathe without assistance. Caregivers are less likely to engage in preventive health behaviours for themselves.

Did you get that last part of the message? I missed it by a fair margin when I was looking after Clair. I slowed down my running regime. Didn't go for a massage as often as I had before. We can only afford so much for health care for the two of us, I told myself. But a lot of the problem for us caregivers reside not just in ignoring preventive health behaviours but in losing the insight that we *need* to do these things for ourselves. We are so busy worrying about our spouses and helping with their care—if not providing it entirely—that we simply forget to look after ourselves. Ironically, this self-neglect often worsens the vicious cycle: we become so tired that we lose insight into our lack of self-care and the factors that are behind it, increasing our lack of self-care even more. In my case, I had at least been going for counselling, and that probably became a factor in delaying my physical collapse until six to eight months after Clair was in the warm, safe, protective hands of Lions Gate Hospital and then the Kiwanis Care Centre (KCC).

Check out what the very helpful Family Caregiver Alliance website has to say about caregiver health, but fasten your seat belt because the site posts a lot of warnings about the roads we have been on, are still on and will likely be travelling for an uncertain time into the future. One article says that research has shown that spousal caregivers who provide thirty-six or more hours per week of care are slightly more likely to smoke and consume more saturated fat. Compared to non-caregivers, women caregivers are twice as likely not to fill a prescription because of the cost (26 versus 13 percent). Nearly three-quarters of caregivers reported that they had not gone to the doctor as often as they should, and more than half had missed appointments with their doctors. Caregivers' self-care also suffers because they lack the time and energy to prepare proper meals or to exercise. Caregivers in rural areas are at an even greater disadvantage for having their own medical needs met due to difficulty getting to a hospital or doctor.

Of 221 caregivers in the baby boomer age range who were surveyed by a Canadian research team in 2010, 35 percent felt their general health had worsened since becoming a caregiver.[3] All of these caregivers reported high levels of fatigue, stress and helplessness as well as depression, but those caregivers who were living with their care recipient were even more vulnerable to negative health effects. Of the 25 caregivers in the study in this category, 60 percent felt their general health had deteriorated since assuming the role of caregiver, and 16 percent of this group reported having experienced suicidal thoughts. Many reported financial burdens and workplace conflicts. (These symptoms were also reported, though to a somewhat lesser extent, by those who were not living with their care recipient.) Is it any wonder that caregivers are sometimes called the invisible second patient?

So what does any of this have to do with you and me? None of these facts and figures would have moved me back in 2004 and 2005 when Clair was first becoming symptomatic. So she had Alzheimer's. That was unfortunate, but I knew we would cope, hang together, see our way through this one day at a time. Caregiver vulnerability? Maybe once in a while, David, I said to myself. But major problems? No, that was something that happened to other people, not to me and certainly not to my patients. That was how I talked to myself then, but I did it quietly so I could not hear my own deceptive words of denial. I pushed the problems away. Lived my life as usual. I was fooling myself, but the biggest deception was my lack of awareness of how *much* I was fooling myself.

In those early days, my conversations with Clair touched on these issues only infrequently because we had more enjoyable things to do together. We did talk—though only in the vaguest of terms—about the future each of us would soon be facing, but part of this talking was encoded with a message of silence. We supported ourselves with an unspoken contract: let us live *only* in the present. We would tip-toe around the important stuff like planning for what was ahead. And as for mental or emotional problems, why, I already had a counsellor, didn't I? She was a darned good one, and Clair was welcome to join us anytime she wanted.

But all the research clearly demonstrates that caregivers like me—and maybe you?—have higher levels of stress than non-caregivers. When caregivers describe themselves, they use words like *frustrated*, *angry*, *drained*, *guilty* and *helpless*, revealing that they are at greater risk for elevated levels of hostility than non-caregivers. They also report having less self-acceptance and feeling less effective and less in control of their lives. Exhausted when they go to bed at night, many of them sleep fitfully, worrying about all the responsibilities awaiting them in the morning. Any one or all of these developments are so important to the caregiver because the physical strain of caring for someone who cannot perform activities of daily living—such as bathing, grooming and toileting—puts them at serious risk for poor physical health outcomes. As a response to the increased stress, many of them drink more or abuse other substances and use prescription and psychotropic drugs more often than non-caregivers.

John, who is caring for his wife at home, described some of his frustrations in dealing with the activities of daily living.

> I'm fortunate that Nancy is very placid, happy most of the time, eats well, sleeps well, is physically healthy, doesn't seem to have agitation, paranoia, anything like that, so we've never had to even think about special medication to quiet her down. But there's this whole scene of trying to get her dressed in the morning . . . if she doesn't want to do it, boy, there's no way she will. You can get a little aggressive with her and she just really tightens up and she's very strong. I quickly learned that I can't push her around. I'm far better off to just let it go by, then go back a half hour later and try again, and she usually does it then with no problem . . . What hasn't helped is my impatience . . . I'm trying *hard* not to

be impatient, but I like order. I like things to be in order and . . .
I like to plan ahead. I like to be organized and you just can't worry
about stuff like that with her. [laughter] In this situation you can't
keep a tight schedule. You can't keep things as neat and tidy as
you might otherwise like.

When I'm away—and I'll be away for a couple of weeks at the
end of the month—I worry about [Nancy's unwillingness to get
into the bathtub]. But last year [the hired care aide] was fairly new
to us, and she looked after Nancy for that period of time, and they
got along fine. Afterwards I said to [the care aide], "How did you
get her in and out of the bathtub?" And it turns out that she just
gets undressed and gets in with her. It's a two-person tub and
she said that seems to help a lot. But I think Nancy has an innate
resistance to showing her body in front of anybody, including me,
and doing it one day doesn't help the next. There's no repetitive
memory there for when she's accepted something that she
will accept it the next hour or the next day, but that's all part of
the disease.

But what's been a real learning exercise is having to get her
to go to the toilet and wipe her bottom and clean her up when
she has an accident. Occasionally she'll get up in the middle of
the night and go to the bathroom, but she sits on the lid so it's a
bit of a mess to clean up the next day. The other day she . . . we
have carpet in our bathroom, unfortunately, and she got up from
having a bowel movement and she's wearing the Depends type
of panties now, and I looked down and it looked as if everything
was okay, but what I hadn't noticed was, I guess, when she stood
up, she dropped a little parcel on the floor and then stepped on
it and walked across the floor, so there were about eight brown
footprints from there to the sink . . . And guess who had to clean
it up? [laughter]

While caregiving can result in a loss of self-identity, lower levels of self-
esteem, constant worry or feelings of uncertainty, one of the most insidious
enemies I struggled with was anxious depression. I am not alone. Estimates
show that between 40 and 70 percent of caregivers have clinically significant symptoms of depression, and somewhere between one-quarter and
one-half of them meet the diagnostic criteria for major depression. Both
my personal and my professional experience has been that depression
increases as the vulnerable partner's condition worsens, compounded by
or interwoven with grief. Unfortunately, research also shows that spousal

caregivers who are at risk of clinical depression and are caring for a spouse with significant cognitive impairment or physical care needs are more likely to engage in harmful behaviour toward their loved one. And sadly enough, both caregiver depression and anxiety often persist, and can even worsen after the partner is placed in a nursing home—as was probably true in my case.

Depression often wields its stealthy, crippling effects in insidious ways that can be masked by alcohol or drug use or abuse. At other times it is expressed in various forms of acting out—rebounding into a new relationship, for example. But we're usually not aware that we *are* depressed until someone points it out to us or we are hit by a depression-related illness such as insomnia—especially early-morning awakening—a lack of energy, suicidal thoughts or a loss of libido. Depression often coexists with anxiety, which may express itself in sleeplessness or agoraphobia (the fear of going out to the market or even just outside the front door). Anxiety may also surface as obsessive–compulsive disorder in the form of unreasonable, bothersome, persistent thoughts or unusual repetitive behaviours (compulsions).

Is loneliness a challenge or obstacle for you as caregiver? I know it has been for me at times since Clair first became symptomatic, even before her AD diagnosis. And it has probably been more so since she went into care. Aloneness—living with oneself, with or without the company of others—is a natural part of the human condition; loneliness, on the other hand, arises when we have difficulty living with our aloneness—that is, as my counsellor reminds me, it is aloneness poorly tolerated. Sometimes I experience aloneness and loneliness together and have difficulty in telling where one stops and the other begins. Little attention has been given to loneliness as a factor in the development of depression in the caregivers of spouses with AD, however. In one research sample, forty-nine AD-caregiving spouses reported significantly higher levels of loneliness and depression than did fifty-two non-caregiving spouses, while AD-caregiving wives reported greater loss of self and significantly higher levels of loneliness and depression than did AD-caregiving husbands.[4] Loneliness was the only predictive variable for AD caregiver depression, explaining 49 percent of the total variance. Therefore, to meet the mental health needs of AD caregiving spouses, it is important that loneliness be addressed along with the development of nursing interventions.

A central, but often overlooked, part of our experience as caregivers is grief, which is often complicated by depression and sometimes also by anxiety. As a caregiver, you may find yourself struggling with grief, though it is sometimes disguised, and it may be difficult, and at times unmanageable or even impossible, to face. The grieving person may be unaware of additional feelings often associated with grief, such as guilt, rumination and resentment, which are almost impossible to share, especially if such feelings have never or rarely been experienced within the partnership. In a study led by Dr. Sara Sanders of the University of Iowa, researchers found that until quite recently most dementia research has overlooked grief among caregivers:

> Seven themes emerged from [this study of] the caregiving experience of individuals with high grief: (a) yearning for the past, (b) regret and guilt, (c) isolation, (d) restricted freedom, (e) life stressors, (f) systemic issues, and (g) coping strategies. The first two themes reflect grief reactions, whereas isolation, restricted freedom, life stressors, and systemic issues possess elements of both grief and caregiver burden and stress. Coping strategies used by this group of caregivers included spiritual faith, social supports and pets. Quantitative analysis confirmed that these themes are unique to individuals with high levels of grief compared with those with moderate/low levels of grief, except for the coping strategies of social support and spiritual faith.[5]

These same researchers found that the caregiver's grief may overlap with depression. This is especially true when the caregiving role comes right on the heels of a previously complicated partnership with unresolved conflicts, mixed feelings, ambivalence, communication difficulties, emotional or physical abuse, or other important yet unresolved issues between the partners. In such cases, the challenge for the caregiving wife is especially acute and the results can be even more detrimental for the caregiver. Dr. Diana B. Denholm, the psychotherapist who wrote *The Caregiving Wife's Handbook* after overseeing her own husband's nightmarish trip through eleven and a half years of multiple illnesses, learned from the wives she interviewed that husbands who were abusive when they were healthy could become veritable tyrants when seriously or terminally ill.

The Alzheimer Society of Canada has prepared a detailed paper on what it terms the "ambiguous loss" that is experienced by most caregivers. This term means loving someone who is there physically, but not present in most other ways, someone who is disappearing in front of our eyes. So what does the caregiver experience in this complicated thing called ambiguous loss? One important aspect of it may be the loss of dreams and unfulfilled expectations in the shared present and the previously fantasized future. In my experience, however, one of the largest and earliest losses I experienced, which occurred soon after Clair's diagnosis, was the disappearance of the shared, communicative partnership that I call *mutuality*. This is that sense that you're on the same page as your partner nine times out of ten. Fighting. Laughing. Making up. There's almost always an agreement to disagree, an understanding that you're with each other (even when briefly you're not with each other) physically, emotionally and psychologically.

The Alzheimer Society of Canada website also makes a useful distinction between *instrumental grievers* and *intuitive grievers*. Instrumental grievers are more comfortable "behaving" their grief, for example, vigorously looking after their loved ones, immersing themselves in projects and services for their living partners, then perhaps busying themselves with memorials for their lost ones. Intuitive grievers, on the other hand, *feel* their grief, often with a wide range of emotions including, but not limited to, sadness, frustration, anger and loneliness. Like most psychological distinctions and differences, of course, there is often an overlap between these two grieving styles within one grieving person.

Ambiguous loss also includes anticipatory grief, letting both the figurative and the actual tears fall before the final loss. With AD, this kind of loss is usually much more prolonged and much more ambiguous than with a partner facing a finite, concrete, major chronic or acute illness with better known, sharper boundaries, both in time and function. As a result, many caregivers of spouses with AD may not receive the acknowledgement or support for their grief that they expect from their families and friends because family and friends don't always realize that the caregiver *is* grieving. On the other hand, because most AD caregivers are aware that the closure of death may be years in the future, they may be unable to address or express their grief while looking after the person and anticipating the losses that still lie ahead. I struggled with the heartbreak of losing Clair day by day, but this breaking-but-not-broken heart was not something my friends would often encourage me to share, explore or ventilate.

Both my personal and my professional experience with grief has been that the bereft often undergo feelings of loss, mourning and sadness on several, often interwoven levels, and these different levels of bereavement will usually reflect the nature of the partnership that preceded the loss. In other words, a simple, uncomplicated yet warm and rewarding relationship will be followed by relatively straightforward grieving, which generally begins long before the physical death of the loved one. The complexity of the "Long Goodbye" of Alzheimer's disease also means suffering from occasional or frequent periods of confusion and perplexity that may resolve themselves before our loved one's physical death occurs.

On the other hand, most relationships have their occasional dark moments with patches of antipathy, anger, frustration or ambivalence that are usually cleanly resolved (although at other times they may be left quietly festering). These dark spots can be expected to pockmark a grieving process that is already complicated by the vagaries, uncertainties and length of the Alzheimer's decline. And where ambivalence lies, we may expect delayed or complicated, difficult experiences of grief and anguish. That is, the bereaved partner will often mourn over the positive partner he/she enjoyed in their time together, but also over the negative experiences that appeared within the span of the relationship. This grief may also be accompanied by relief that the bleaker side of the partnership has come to an end, though at the same time these feelings of respite, relief and release are often associated with feelings of guilt and sadness and may begin long before the Alzheimer's partner's physical death occurs. Finally, the bereaved one may experience—silently and even unconsciously—the regret, the wistful fantasies and the broken heart for the positive, perhaps idealized, partnership that he/she was cheated of by the Alzheimer's diagnosis: the partnership that never was.

All these levels of grief may be interwoven and overlapping. While we miss so much those warm and positive experiences of our lost partnership, we may find ourselves grieving over—though at the same time celebrating the cessation of—the gloomier, shadier areas of our now imperfect match. And finally, often quietly, we may find ourselves wondering why we didn't have the ideal relationship we had dreamed of, or the kind our parents or our friends had—or that we thought they had. All of these elements can make grief subjectively, inordinately complicated and painful, but avoiding the necessary steps along the paths of bereavement may exact an even sharper, steeper price in our future with ourselves, and with others.

|||||||||||||||||||||||||||||||

All my reading and experience as a psychotherapist indicate that female caregivers (who make up about two-thirds of all unpaid caregivers) fare worse than their male counterparts. They have higher levels of depressive and anxiety symptoms and lower levels of subjective well-being, life satisfaction and physical health than male caregivers. At the same time, women will set the bar higher, sometimes significantly so, spending more energy, more heart, mind, body and soul, in looking after a loved one than men will, while working harder to take care of themselves. In fact, although statistics tell us that women are twice as likely as men to get Alzheimer's as they age (in fact, in Canada in 2013, women represented 72 percent of cases, according to the Alzheimer Society of Canada), within most AD caregivers' support groups there are twice as many women as men, a ratio that one might expect to be reversed. This ratio means women as a whole take their caregiving and caretaking assignments, fantasies, needs and desires more seriously than men do. The upside is that the object of a woman's caregiving is likely to have a better life for her efforts. However, the downside is that, on average, women are more likely to pay a physical or emotional price for their commitment to a loved one struggling with AD or dementia.

One study of twenty wives caring for spouses with dementia describes their experiences as a process of "interpretive caring."[6] The women in the study began the process either by seeing changes in their husbands or by recognizing changes in their work. After accepting these changes, they gradually began taking over their husbands' roles and responsibilities, rewriting identities for their husbands that incorporated the dementia and rewriting identities for themselves to reflect their new roles, abilities and strengths. The wives eventually set about constructing a new daily life to sustain both themselves and their partners. This process is neutral and allows for positive aspects of caring to be considered along with grief and frustration.

In one of my interviews for this book, Margaret, a recently bereaved caregiver, described how she experienced the process of gradually assuming a new role.

> Donald loved doing the cryptic crossword, and he used to say that when he did the crossword and he finished it, it meant that his mind was still working. So when he stopped, it was very upsetting to him, but he just said, "I can't do this anymore." He recognized that his brain couldn't make the connections that were needed to complete the crossword. The other thing he stopped was doing the bills. He used to handle all the bills; he would write the cheques, put them in the envelopes, take them to the post office. And then gradually I helped him with them, and I would stand over him, and I'd say, "Okay, this is the Hydro bill, it is one hundred and twenty-nine dollars and sixty-three cents, now you put the date up here. What's today's date?" And he would put it in, he was doing the writing. And then one day he said, "I can't do this anymore." All the way through he would recognize when it came time to give something up. And so I took over doing the bills.

Nora experienced the same role change but also enlisted the help of her daughter in resolving the problems she encountered.

> Because Sam is a controller, he handled all the money, but as he lost control, I tried to loosen his grip a little, and he was resentful. But I did it slowly, and then our daughter set it all up for me online, so now I don't have to worry about forgetting to pay a bill. Sam still gets a pile of letters every day from all these charitable

organizations because that's his big interest—giving away money to charities. But I had to explain to him that it wasn't right to give his Mastercard number to outfits like this over the phone, and I finally got him to stop doing that.

For caregivers, the significance of the research and statistics is plain: making changes must be factored into your lifestyle early in the progress of the disease. In my own case, it was only with considerable hindsight that I realized that since Clair's diagnosis I had unconsciously been constructing a program that would help me run toward the answers rather than away from the questions. First, it came to me that I needed to slow down and catch my breath. Zen Buddhists remind us, "Don't just do something. Stand there." So I prayed and meditated. Then after a time I began attending a co-ed support group for those with partners or parents living with AD; less often I visited another group for husbands whose wives had Alzheimer's. Groups of this kind are the most logical, safest places to go to unburden your fears, hopes and guilt, get non-judgemental support and benefit from the experiences shared by others—their trials and errors, memories of disappointment, anguish and grief. At the same time, you can share your own feelings of triumph, closure and satisfaction in enduring and overcoming—the results of your hard work, patience and courage.

For most of the caretakers I met there, the group has been a lifeline. For my friend Margaret, it was a surprise to find such support. She told me,

> This support group is so important because when you first go there, you think, Oh, nobody will understand. [laughter] How can they? I'm going through this by myself. I mean, who else could feel this way? And then you realize they're *all* experiencing the same thing that you are, you know? That's why the support group is so good. It was certainly a huge, huge help.

Nora was fortunate to find a weekly support group that includes activities for the spouses with memory loss, but the caregivers from that group also meet separately.

> Once a month we have a session that is just for caregivers— discussion time. Most of the same caregivers are there, but there are others as well. One woman told me that her husband wouldn't come [to the weekly group] because he says there's absolutely nothing wrong with him. I think I'm very, very lucky to be in the group I'm in—and the others in the group feel the same way. We're quite cohesive, very helpful to one another, and the organizers are slowly adding others who can benefit from

that. Our partners are still at the stage where they're mobile and still at home, so [the organizers] can bring in others with bigger problems [than we have].

One lady told us everything that was going wrong in her house, and we gave her most of one session, and then she told us how her husband had always sunbathed in the nude on their sailboat, but now [the boat] was in their backyard, and he was still sunbathing in the nude on the sailboat, horrifying all the neighbours. And we laughed so hard we almost fell off our chairs, and by this time she's laughing too. So this was the perfect medicine for her. If you could just see the difference in her! This is the third time she's been [to the group] and if you could just see her face! At first she would come in and just sit there like *this*, and now she's in there with the best of them, telling stories and getting feedback. Getting support.

A woman whose husband is going downhill very fast apologized after her second session with us. She said, "I'm terribly sorry to be dumping on you people like this because my situation is so much worse than yours, and it must be very downing for you." But it wasn't. We feel very supportive of her, and there are too many of us that are upbeat that one person can't bring us down. (I went to one of the courses that the AD Society gives, and *that* was a downer!) I think if I was giving other caregivers advice, I'd say check very carefully the make-up of the support group.

Insight is our big friend during these times, and it can be gathered from a support group, a really good counsellor or psychotherapist, or from friends or family. I am fortunate to have several supportive and interested friends and family members (from both Clair's family and my own) who will meet me for breakfast to talk about my concerns. Most often the conversation with them begins with "How's Clair?" but this question is only the beginning; it's an invitation to share more deeply. It is also an opening for me to encourage family members—and friends—to come out, to open up. What helped several us in my extended family was attending Kerri Sutherland's six-month-long, family-oriented seminar series on dementia. Kerri, the Support and Education Coordinator for the Alzheimer Society of B.C. (North Shore Division), is a good, unsentimental teacher and led us through the emotional, medical, spiritual and physical labyrinth that is central to the Alzheimer's experience.

I used to wonder about the people I saw out walking or waiting for the elevator in my apartment building, each of them with a small Jack Russell, pug or dachshund on a leash. Then one day it came to me: they've found companionship, and companionship is exactly what is missing in the caregiver's life. We *all* need somebody or something nearby. For you as a caregiver, this might mean acquiring a pet. But if you are not a dog or cat person, it could mean making one or two new human friendships that oscillate between warmth and heat. If you are enjoying these new friendships and are sleeping well in the meantime, you are probably doing something right. (And it's okay to flirt or be a little coy with the opposite sex if that's your style).

It took a while, but slowly I began to take better care of my physical self. After Clair was admitted to KCC, in spite of a history of atrial fibrillation and Prinzmetal's angina (a condition mimicking a heart attack but without actual heart damage), I had fallen into the habit of not exercising as much as I had been. Previously I had run in the Vancouver Sun's 10K race several times, and in 2008 and 2009 I had cycled the Seattle to Portland bike race, but as Clair became sicker and I began to devote more time to taking care of her, I ran less and didn't cycle at all. Then one evening in January 2013 as I waited at the bus stop after a warm visit with Clair, I started to curse the cold weather. Then I thought, Why don't you walk a little bit, David . . . you know, just up to that lamppost and back? And so I did, and with a longer-than-usual wait for my bus, I was able to do seventeen cycles to the lamppost and back. Then just for fun, I estimated the distance—135 feet each way or 270 feet per cycle. Using my calculator the next morning, I discovered I had walked almost seven-eighths of a mile—just while waiting for the bus! That was a lot more fun than standing there by myself cursing the cold or the rain, and it was much better for my heart too. What would you rather be doing, I asked myself, walking or cursing? And I found myself remembering that if it's good for the heart, it's good for the head. So I started running again and walking longer distances, like making the climb from the Phibbs Bus Exchange all the way up the hill to KCC to visit Clair rather than taking the bus.

This need for exercise was reinforced when I talked to Margaret, who was emphatic about the value to caregivers of keeping physically active.

> Exercise is terribly important to every caregiver. You need to keep up your physical energy levels. I study Pilates—it's just a small group. And I also have a horse so I ride each and every day. I used to call him my therapy horse because I would go and visit him and I would feel better. I would see him in the morning and then visit Donald in the afternoon, and it kind of gave me a leg up. It made me calm and ready to deal with Donald's needs.

Nowadays I watch my diet. I decided to lose a few pounds, even though my anxious friends insisted, "You don't need to lose weight, David!" And I began going for massages again. Massage is a reminder to yourself that you still have a body, one worthy of nurturance and TLC. Once during a layover at the Seattle airport, I paid for a drop-in massage, right there in front of hundreds of travellers. Previously I had laughed at the "vanity" of people who exercised this indulgence in airports. But not this time, and am I glad I did it! That massage was a treat for myself.

With the help of Molly, the therapist and counsellor I have been seeing for over ten years, I began dealing with the issues surrounding my chronic anxiety, slowly learning how to separate my own anxiety from my friends' caring anxiety about me and Clair and our medical and physical health. These changes saw me become—again slowly—less anxious about my own anxiety (a condition also known as meta-anxiety, or a feeling about a feeling). In the process I began to identify and appreciate others' anxiety about me—however well-meaning—and to distance myself from their over-identifying with me or Clair. I developed better boundaries and a sense of where they stopped and I began, which meant less anxiety and more self-awareness for me—and probably for my friends and family members, too.

Finally—and this is one hundred percent hindsight—even though Clair was in a care home and was gradually drifting away from me, I refused to write off what we had shared. She and I began a series of trial-and-error experiments in how to stay in touch with each other. What did we have to lose? Nothing! And as hard as I could be on myself, Clair was very forgiving. If I goofed somehow or was clumsy in trying to connect with her, she would often just laugh—and within a few hours (or, more recently, a few minutes) probably also forget. It was a stretch, but I became a kinder person than I had been in the past. Though never a blue meanie, I had no idea how much more fun I would have being even kinder with her, as together we began experimenting with new ways to be together in a virtually risk-free environment.

My counsellor Molly has helped me experience, understand and to some extent sort through the complicated grief that follows when AD visits a marriage or partnership. Operating as my research assistant, she gives me support and feedback, and though unable to answer all the questions I am struggling with, she helps me to sharpen the questions.

So what is the message in this chapter? Get help. I had done so after my late wife, Betsy, succumbed to cancer, both for my kids and for myself. I had to seek help again when I was losing Clair in the more disjointed, fragmented, now-you-see-her, now-you-don't fashion consistent with an Alzheimer's diagnosis. If you are stuck in this place, talk with friends or family whom you trust and feel comfortable with. But think also about getting grief counselling coordinated with visiting a counsellor, psychologist or a psychiatrist with whom you feel comfortable. And don't hesitate to do some window-shopping until you find the one or two professionals who understand your situation, who treat you with warm respect and with whom you feel comfortable, respected, hopeful, helpful and encouraged.

||||||||||||||||||||||||||||||||

All these previews of what might happen to you come with an enormous silver lining, one that is quite difficult to appreciate when you are under the cloud of losing a beloved. But we need to understand that, in meeting and surmounting these obstacles, we also grow, often in unexpected ways and sometimes marvellously, as in the notion that what doesn't destroy us makes us stronger. Of course, this sentiment is difficult to appreciate when we are going through trial and torment. It is helpful to know that in Chinese, the concept of crisis is written as two characters, one meaning a time of danger, the other a time of opportunity. It *is* a crisis, or a series of overlapping or intersecting crises, that you and I are, have been or will be experiencing.

The eloquent words of Rabbi Sincha Kling have provided enormous comfort for me as he has voiced what I struggled with but could not articulate myself. These words come from a *Yizkor*, or memorial service.

> When my loved one is taken from me, shall I mourn?
> When my dear one departs forever,
> Shall I wail and rend my flesh as I do my garment?
> No! That is not the way.
>
> I may find the road ahead lonely.
> I may dread tomorrow without that voice, without
>   that smile.
> I may not know whence will come the courage to continue.
> Yet I shall not despair!
>
> I will refuse to become bitter over what I shall lack.
> When my loved one leaves me, I shall indeed shed tears.
> Yet, even then, I shall utter a hymn—
> A song of joy for what has been.
>
> Barukh Atah Adonai!
> Praised are You, O God!
> You have allowed me to know love;
> You have granted me an eternal treasure.

CHAPTER SEVEN

Sexuality and Intimacy

I was feeling as if I was the only lonely, horny person in my crowd, among my friends, even among the women and men within my Alzheimer's caregivers' support group. Could it be, I asked myself, that I am the only one haunted by thoughts and dreams of sexual intimacy, consumed with memories of the wonderful intimacy I had experienced with both Betsy and Clair? The only one with fantasies of re-experiencing it? Or is it just that I am the only one who needs to talk about such things? (A friend teased me, "Kirkpatrick, you are *incorrigible!*")

But it turns out I wasn't the only one. I was quite relieved to discover *Sexuality and the Alzheimer's Patient* by E.L. Ballard and C. Poer. Although the book was published back in 1993, the conditions they wrote about have not changed much since then. In a section on coping with changes in intimate relationships between caregivers and their spouses with long-term chronic illnesses, the authors note that physicians seem reluctant to address the question of how those relationships change. For example, one seventy-six-year-old man who was caring for his wife with dementia told them that no doctor had ever asked him about his marriage or sexuality although it played a large part in his well-being.

Although dementia is an age-related disorder, no one can tell you or me how much intimacy, sexuality and their associated pleasures and conflicts could be and should be related to age. A psychotherapy patient who is looking after a very ill spouse asked me just the other day, "David, I want to get laid so badly . . . but do you think at sixty-five I'm too old for that?" My only answer was, "And what book did you read that in?" Only *you* can gauge how much your sexual relationship, along with the emotional and physical intimacy within your partnership, has meant to you and how much the persistent memories of those intimate times together remind you, encourage you, urge you and inspire you to continue searching for special moments in your relationship now. Ballard and Poer noted that at a conference sponsored by the Caregiver Resource Centers of California in 1992, the keynote presentation on sexuality and intimacy featured a panel of caregivers who were asked by the moderator if anyone had ever asked them how the disease had affected their ability to be intimate. Each panel member responded that the subject had never come up with any professional, not even in a caregiver support group. In fact, our society as a whole tends to deny the sexuality of sick people and older people, as well as their need for closeness, while at the same time denying the sexuality and need for intimacy of the *partners* of those same people.[1]

This subject came up in my interview with John, whose wife had been diagnosed with Alzheimer's disease eight years earlier but who recently became confused about her relationship to him. He told me,

> After a while what I started to notice was—and what I missed the most—was the intimacy, which kind of dropped off. She's very affectionate in terms of wanting to cuddle and hugs and that sort of thing, but anything beyond that. . . At one point I was approaching her in bed and trying to get some activity going, and she just said, "No. John wouldn't like this. You know, I hardly know you . . ."
>
> And that was pretty hurtful. I backed off right away, of course. So apart from that, what I've missed, I think, over these years is the lack of companionship, the fact that I can't really talk to her about anything significant. At the end of the day we used to sit over dinner and talk about our day and who we saw and what we did, and that has no meaning for her anymore. It's just that she doesn't absorb any of it, you know?

For Graham, the end of intimacy was more abrupt. When I commented that caring for his wife at home had perhaps allowed for more physical contact between them, he said that there had not been much of that. He explained:

> [Before she died] I hadn't slept in the same bedroom with Yvonne for many years . . . right from the time she woke up in the night and turned over and said, "Who the hell are you?" And I said, "It's just me, Yvonne. It's Graham."

"Get out of my house!"

And I said, "Well, I'll just go in the other room, Yvonne." But she continued to be afraid. She walked out into the kitchen and came back with a butcher knife *this* long, and she said, "Get out of my house!" And when I refused, she went crazy. She said, "I'm going to kill you!" She said that many times. Ultimately I took the knife away from her, and I just abandoned the idea of sleeping in the same room and left her there by herself. That's not to say that some nights I didn't go in and lie down beside her. Lots of nights I did. Some nights it was okay, but other nights it was, "Who are you?" And then I quickly exited . . . She didn't know what she was doing, she was afraid, that's all. She didn't know who I was. The first time I didn't know what was happening because how can [your wife] be afraid of you? I mean, I've lived with Yvonne for forty-five years. How could she be afraid of me?

Nobody has any idea what's going to happen with this disease or where you're going to go. Absolutely no one.

The phenomenon that both these men encountered in their relationship with their AD-afflicted wives is known as Capgras syndrome, the so-called delusion of doubles, in which the individual becomes convinced that her/his partner is *not really* her/his partner but someone masquerading as that person. Studies suggest that about 10 percent of those with Alzheimer's will develop Capgras syndrome, usually in the middle or later phases of the disease.[2] Listening to Graham and John describe their experiences, I couldn't help but remember how Clair had become agitated a few years earlier at a yoga class because "David might find out about us." This was followed by her anxiety on a trip to Oregon, when she asked how we would tell David about our affair, and then by the heartbreaking episodes when she phoned the police to report a stranger (me) in her house. Wondering whether she still harboured that belief, I tried a different tack one afternoon in late 2013 when I visited her. Rather than reminding her as usual that I was David, as we sat down on one side of the large foyer of Cypress Cove East to chat, I said, "Honey, I've got good news!" She seemed somewhat interested, maybe even curious.

"David couldn't make it," I continued, "but he was glad I was seeing you today because he knows how much I care for you, too. He loves you a whole bunch! And so do I! So I asked David if it was okay for you and me to snuggle. But he told me, 'Only if it's okay with Clair!' And that made sense to me!" I began lightly caressing her back.

We went to her room where we did a slow, silent dance without Clair moving her feet. Afterwards I flopped down on her bed, but for the first time she did not lie down beside me, even with her feet on the floor. So I got up, took her hand and led her to a chair where we could talk more. And then she surprised me by caressing my left upper inner thigh as she had not done in fifteen months or more. Aroused, I watched her hands tenderly stroke my thigh, but she stopped there. I wasn't sure if my revelation had made an impression, but she *seemed* to be intrigued by the idea and maybe even comfortable being with me in David's absence.

|||||||||||||||||||||||||||||||||

For most couples coping with dementia, physical intimacy continues to be a rich source of mutual comfort, support and pleasure for many years after diagnosis, but the effects of Alzheimer's are not predictable. Some people with dementia seem to lose interest in sex at a very early stage, and while they may receive reassurance from being stroked, hugged or cuddled, they are no longer able to initiate any affection themselves. Consider the case of my old high school friend, Jane, who is bravely navigating the steps and (only occasional) missteps of looking after her AD husband at home, continuing to seek love, asking for hugs from him. It is a wrenching experience. She writes:

> I just can't imagine it when we no longer can share a bed or a kitchen. Those places are the centres of our life, where we share all our feelings, the heart of our lives. The everyday things are the most precious. I hate to think of John sleeping somewhere alone, eating alone.
>
> And for me, thinking I won't be touched again—or almost never. As if someone put a sheet of glass between us . . . How many times has my heart stopped racing when I felt the touch of John's hand, how many times has just curling up beside him in bed centred me? Made the world seem right in the midst of very wrong?
>
> We've been married thirty-four years. His presence is calming for me, even now when he is impaired. Just the presence of his body, so familiar to me, is calming. Doctors, too, say that in controlled tests, that is so. His face lights up with a big smile, still, when he sees me, too. To lose this, to reach a time when he doesn't know me, I wonder how will I stand it? Often I wish he'd just put his arms around me. But he forgets how now. I have to ask him for a hug. I have to say, "John, I need a hug. Will you put your arms around me and give me a hug?" Then he does and we both stop a minute and enjoy it.

Speaking of stopping for a minute . . . John takes so long and is so deliberate in what he's doing now, especially with his clothes and his "special" pocket belongings—often a pocket knife, a toothpick, a penny and a napkin—that it makes me nuts. I want to hurry him up so I can take him to wherever we're going at the moment. And yet at other times I'm learning to experience the moment again from him because he's like a child. We were sitting in the living room and he saw a rainbow outside over the water. He got up from his chair and walked right outside to see. And then so did I. He's pointed out clouds and rabbits and children to me, too. And I look.

Then a few days later Jane wrote to tell me of another incident in her life with John. She had hurt her back and added,

Then, because he was concerned, he said, "What can I do?"

And I said, "Give me a back rub. I love to feel your hands on me."

I do. Even though he's battling AD, it's still so comforting to me. I can't bear to think there will be a time when his hands won't touch me anymore. And no one's will. It will be unbearably lonely. And you know, as he rubbed lotion on my back, as he finished one area, he would cover it up so I wouldn't be cold. It touched me so that he remembered that. He had always done that.

I think my awareness is painfully heightened.

Unfortunately, many Alzheimer's support groups shy away from conversations about sexuality. Graham, who describes himself as "highly organized and very much in control," felt the need for such discussions, but was warned off by the group's facilitator who "tiptoed around the topic." She felt it was more important to provide what Graham described as

advice as to what we should be careful for, about how single guys after their wives die are rare commodities. That we should be very careful who we associate with because there will be lots of ladies to choose from and lots of them that will be interested in us. And she started giving us a lecture . . . So many men, she said, have to have somebody in their bed every night. They have to have that, it's just essential for them, and those guys just fall into bed with the first female that comes along. And I thought, Man oh man, who's she to be giving us this lecture? She's a nice lady, but . . . [laughter].

As I look back over the first fifteen months that Clair spent at the Kiwanis Care Centre (KCC), I see that she was not the only one making adjustments, learning new routines and procedures and finding new rhythms. I would visit her every other day, at first usually greeted by a surprised but pleased look on her face and sometimes a comment such as "I thought you'd never get here!" And while often taking advantage of our beautiful weather and going for a walk in the nearby woods, my first instincts would be to hug her warmly, then take her by the hand and lead her back to her room with its single but not unmanageable bed for quiet cuddling. Often but not always, I would tip my hand and tell her what I was looking forward to. And she would smile, heading straight to her room holding my hand. Almost every visit saw us connecting—me holding her, caressing and stroking her arms and face while she closed her eyes beneath her omnipresent glasses with a warm and contented smile on her face. Occasionally I would sing softly to her. The words from the Irving Berlin musical *Call Me Madam* were almost guaranteed to elicit a smile or a chuckle from her.

I found myself practising skills I possessed only at intermediate levels: warmth, quietness, tenderness and surrender. Afterwards, as I let myself out and headed for my bus, I would feel incredibly fortunate to be in love and experiencing mutuality again. And I reminded myself that love is to tenderness as wine is to brandy.

It was somewhere around August 2011—six months after she entered KCC—that I began reflecting more deeply on the nature of the marriage that Clair and I now shared. I could see even then that both the depth and breadth of our love were dissolving. There were good reasons for this. We no longer shared a home or a bed. We no longer shopped together, nor did we talk about shopping together, or even spend a few minutes discussing our shopping list. "Didn't we just have salmon three days ago? How about cheese fondue tonight? Sure, it's labour intensive but . . ." Conversations like these had gone out the door along with the mutuality that allowed us to cuss and discuss, to argue, disagree, then usually but not always reconcile or compromise on some point in our day-to-day discourse. And often laugh about it, too!

The unspoken intimacy and tenderness between us, both in and out of our shared queen-sized bed, had at first sharply diminished, then just plain disappeared along with mutuality as the AD bleached out Clair's personality, her memory and her vocabulary. It would eventually destroy even her dynamic, vivacious essence. From our first meeting I had admired Clair for her strength, her spunk and her assertiveness. There had also been a comforting yet important balance between her kind of strength and mine, but as I had to take more responsibility for her medical decisions, this balance also faded.

I saw her questions, curiosity and interest in her children and mine diminish sharply, seemingly replaced by her own deep hurts, areas of grief and longing. I was greeted less often with statements like, "Robert [her son] phoned me this morning!" as her memory loss robbed her of these precious moments. Instead, more and more often she made announcements such as, "Hugh was here this morning!" But Hugh, her beloved older brother, had met his death by drowning over twenty years earlier in a body surfing accident in Hawaii. This and similar comforting memories seemed to be filling the vacuums within her cognitive bank, replacing her awareness of the here and now.

By default, I was becoming the stronger one in our loving partnership, the one responsible for making things happen, for making decisions affecting one or both of us, without being able to consult openly with Clair and without having the benefit of her strength and wisdom. At the same time, "making things happen" was becoming a smaller and smaller task as Clair's living location, caregivers, diet, menu, dress and recreation were all clustered at KCC. I was left with decisions such as where in the woods we would walk that day or the choice of Depends for her (for the latter decisions the KCC nursing staff relied on me as if I were Clair's father). I felt somewhat marginalized there because it wasn't my home. And so the degree of overlap that characterizes most intimate relationships and marriages ebbed away steadily from month to month. Caregiving and caretaking were slowly replacing the caring for each other that is the milieu in which mutuality thrives.

But my perspective was about to widen and deepen further. One Monday morning in late September 2011, several weeks after Clair's seventieth birthday, I began reflecting on the way our love life—or more precisely our sex life and most poignantly our lovemaking life—had slowed to a halt since her Alzheimer's diagnosis some four years earlier. This had been especially true in the last two years, but even more sharply since her move into KCC. Intellectually I understood why things had come pretty much to a stop. At least I thought I understood. It was because one of the sharpest setbacks, as well as one of the first losses with Clair's Alzheimer's disease, had been that loss of mutuality within our relationship. Added to this was simply the loss of time together. For a while, her absence was enough to sharpen my appetite to lie closely with her, although I was never sure what it was like for her. But after a time, while it was not exactly a turn-off, I found that less intimacy with her also meant less of a relationship.

Now on this September day I found myself asking how our lack of emotional and sexual intimacy affected Clair. It didn't seem fair to me that she was deprived of that wonderfully warm closeness that had previously characterized our relationship while at the same time her recent memory was being so brutally stripped away from her. We would still go for walks in the woods near KCC, holding hands, at times with our arms entwined around each other. We hugged often and kissed warmly and tenderly, although I have to admit this was usually initiated by me (though rarely if ever refused by Clair). We exchanged vows of *I love you!* or variations on that theme, and I never doubted the sincerity of the words, no matter which partner voiced them. But what I missed more than the kisses or the sex was the lovemaking, the tenderness that had accompanied our sexual encounters in those earlier times, the closeness and the intimacy that followed surrender. And the surrender itself had always been made safe by Clair—and over time, maybe by me, too. There is little or no intimacy without surrender, and there is rarely surrender without safety.

In Barry Peterson's wonderful memoir *Jan's Story*, a tale that began before his beloved wife's Alzheimer's diagnosis, I read of Peterson's conflict over a similar issue. Sarah Polley's movie *Away from Her*, starring Julie Christie and Gordon Pinsent, also brings out the underlying conflict between sexuality and closeness within an Alzheimer's marriage. But neither the book nor the movie provided a blueprint for what I wanted to know now: how does one experience, enjoy and maintain both heat and warmth in a loving relationship when one partner has a serious, progressive, debilitating illness affecting his/her cognition, memory and judgement, an illness that pushes the partners farther and farther apart, at first emotionally, then intellectually and psychologically, and eventually separates them physically?

Just two days later, while I was on my way to KCC, a possible additional conflict for both of us hit me: with her AD, it was possible that Clair could not say no to me. And that wasn't fair either. That insight or awareness was followed by an increased sense of closeness to Clair the next day, though I had no idea why, nor did I spend time reflecting on it. But now I had mixed feelings about that closeness, and this was foremost in my mind as I led Clair into her bedroom, lay down on her bed and after softening the lights, spooned with her, her back nestled to my abdomen. I felt more aroused than I had been in months. In caressing her, I could tell that the nursing aides had not helped her put on her bra that day. I wanted to stroke her right breast, the one remaining after her left mastectomy for breast cancer some two and a half decades earlier.

Then returning to my thoughts from the previous day, choosing my words slowly and cautiously as I held her, I said, "You know, Clair . . . you can say no or yes or maybe or maybe not or . . . anything you want to say!"

She responded slowly and softly, but also quite clearly. "I think . . . not right now." And then she was quiet.

"Would you like to say more, honey?" I queried.

"Well . . . there are a lot of people out there," she said, gesturing toward her door. "And I'm with them . . . every day."

"So . . . it's kind of like a . . . uh . . . like a . . . privacy issue, eh?" I offered quietly.

"Yes."

If she said more, I missed it or didn't remember it when I was writing about this visit in my journal a day later. I continued to hold her quietly, still feeling close to her, and told her how much she meant to me.

Returning to our apartment, I mused over how much she had taught me that day. Privacy had probably not been the essential issue. Instead, she had been communicating her new discomfort in loving me in our old ways. Of course, love is not sex and sex is not love, but because sexuality and loving had been so intimately interwoven into the first twelve to fourteen years of our relationship, I had unconsciously and continuously taken their one-ness for granted without further thinking or ever discussing it with Clair.

But now as her own emotional responses—with or without me—were becoming more and more difficult for me to decipher, I was freer to concentrate on my loving her. Which I did. But the opportunity Clair had inadvertently given the two of us that day dawned on me very, very slowly. On some visits I missed it completely, but more often I was somewhat aware of the chance to love her deeply, intimately and unconditionally without the need for sex between us. And on my very best days I fully absorbed this chance. It was a new experience, and on these days I always felt myself walking out of KCC to my bus stop with my footsteps on air.

A second problem at this time revolved around my occasional low self-esteem. Would she remember this lovemaking without sex the next day? And did that make a difference? Was I perhaps struggling with my own inner fears of Clair forgetting me entirely? Or the even greater fear of our marriage being lost within her progressively under-functioning memory bank? At times like these, I remembered my friends telling me to "live in the moment." This was no longer a cliché, and if I really listened carefully to those four words, they were a challenge, an opportunity and a gift. Today I can see that my eagerness and willingness to live in the moment now came from the gift of courage that all of us with an Alzheimer's partner have access to—and that, quite possibly, on some level our partners have access to as well.

Rich O'Boyle, the author of "Intimacy, Marriage and Alzheimer's Disease," writes warmly and wisely about sexuality and dementia, noting the many differences and points of tension that arise in a partnership with a demented spouse. Memory gaps, impulsive behaviour, medication side-effects and suspiciousness—all these and more may mark the trail into our later years, O'Boyle notes, but he adds that understanding behaviours in these terms "depersonalizes" the impact.[3]

O'Boyle's words weave nicely with those of Ballard and Poer, who point out that our sexual relationships with our partners have many aspects that overlap in unpredictable but often warm and pleasing ways. I was happily reminded of this after one very tender visit and walk with Clair—this was more than two years since we had last enjoyed sexual intercourse—and I felt a oneness with her that superseded any attempt to analyze or understand it. Did she experience the same or similar feelings? At the time I sensed that she did. My point here is the importance of exploring and experimenting with your partner, seeking old and new wavelengths of connectedness. Listen to your intuition, to your feelings, without spending time trying to analyze the wonder of it all. Enjoy what each of you, both of you, have discovered, separately and together, reinforcing something old, something new. In other words, have fun together. Live in the moment.

I felt less lonely, less alone and more comforted in my continuing efforts to stay in intimate contact with Clair after I read a study based on another couple's efforts to find different forms of contact to nurture the intimacy so badly disrupted by AD. British clinical psychologist Les Todres and nursing professor Kathleen Galvin looked at the coping strategies one husband relied on to keep in touch with his wife in great phenomenological—that is, subjective, sensory and experiential—detail.[4] As the caring experience developed and changed for the husband, the authors identified six stages in the relationship: first he had to learn to live with her memory loss; second, he gradually adjusted to the more limited horizons in their life together; third, he demonstrated his caring in more practical ways; fourth, he adjusted to the changed level of intimacy; fifth, he accepted living apart; and sixth, he accepted his role as his wife's advocate.

This husband and wife reconnected with each other by bridging the gap between physical caregiving and more intimate relating that stopped short of full sexuality. The result was that the opportunities for physical intimacy continued and became more directly intimate (kissing and cuddling). Such moments of physical intimacy and skin-to-skin contact also functioned as a background feeling that broke through the struggles of control and resistance between them in their increasingly disparate and fixed roles.

After Clair entered the care home, she and I had connected with four primary languages: snuggling, kissing, music and laughter. After a year the snuggling had worn thin, but we both continued to enjoy kissing tenderly. Music remained a connection, and laughter was as strong as ever. I was able to get a chuckle, even a laugh, from her each time I returned to a familiar anecdote from our sexual lovemaking days, when I had relished a ritual in which I would kiss each of her ten toes. Toes being neither public nor private, they succeeded in bridging the gap between the two, something I was by then more conscious of in my physical partnership with Clair. You might call it foreplay or a procedure or a tradition, yet our twenty toes seemed to have had a mind of their own, enjoying each other's company while never keeping us apart. And the dialogue I recalled from those days was still guaranteed to elicit a chortle or a giggle from Clair. It went something like this:

CLAIR: But David, you don't know where my feet have been!

DAVID: I don't know and I don't care!

Then together we would laugh. And I remembered those tender, special moments when I penned a poem celebrating her toes—and mine. It began like this:

I miss my wife in care and remind her when I kiss her toes
That there are at least five double dates here, I do suppose.
And counting all continents there are probably for a start
Something like maybe seventy billion of these small
    functional works of art.

With our partners wrestling with Alzheimer's or some other form of dementia, it behooves us to search out and explore new forms of intimacy, including but not limited to the affectionate silliness, tenderness and reverence outlined in the above poem. To do this, we must analyze the challenges as well as the possible rewards of not running away from our dismay and separateness from our loved ones, but *toward* them on as many pathways as possible and finding the many potential answers to our discomfort and apprehension.

Tuning into Clair and her particular needs became a rewarding experience for me, though often a stretch as well. The day in September 2011 when I finally understood that I no longer enjoyed her consent for making sexual love was a real learning occasion for me. All of us with an AD-afflicted spouse have to learn about performance and awkwardness as we reconnect (or *attempt* to reconnect) with a partner who is not the same partner that we once knew—one, in fact, who is becoming a quite different person on an unpredictable timetable. What had been harder for me to visualize and appreciate was that I was *also* a different person, that when Clair had phoned the RCMP to report a stranger within our house, she wasn't entirely delusional. Although she was different, I was also becoming different—a sadder, lonelier and certainly more anxious person.

For Clair and me, however, there was still more than one or two silver linings to our Alzheimer's cloud. Tenderness was one. I could not tell how she felt about warmth by then, but I know my appreciation of the warmth I experienced between us at that time had increased, not only physically but especially emotionally. And I know that I was less inhibited in reminding her how much she meant to me as well as how much I missed her, an example of how we can voice sincere emotions with our loved ones in words that are not only genuine but also not hurtful. Had I voiced these feelings with her five or ten years earlier? Sometimes—but in neither the quantity nor the quality that I enjoyed sharing with her later.

I am, I think, much more sharply tuned to issues today that I never thought much about before, perhaps because those issues—love, children, loss, longing and appreciation, for example—had never or rarely surfaced in the days before AD entered our lives. And one of the most important of those issues was the communication of consent. Although Clair could no longer say no to me, that did *not* mean that she no longer had feelings regarding sexual intimacy, closeness or tenderness, and it was up to me to recognize, validate and appreciate her feelings. And so our relationship, its texture and its nuances, continued to evolve even as our verbal discourse— especially on Clair's part—devolved.

Quality Dementia Care: Understanding Dementia Care and Sexuality in Residential Facilities, published by Alzheimer's Australia, cautions readers not to look for easy solutions within these powerful, dynamic changes and challenges.[5] This booklet reminds those of us experiencing intimacy conflicts with a partner struggling with dementia to be patient and avoid arbitrary answers or solutions. They point out that sexual expression without a loss of dignity or self-esteem must be balanced with human rights and duty of care. These words were very meaningful to me as I searched for ways to reach both *in* to and *out* to Clair. As the days went by, though, the cues and feedback from her often, but not always, became hazier. From hugging and holding her to kissing the top of her head, I continued to seek some way— *any* way—to connect. Sometimes it was by sharing memories of earlier, more clear-cut times of closeness, kindness, mischief and laughter. Even talking dirty would sometimes get a chortle from her—a source of joy to me as laughter was gradually becoming one of the few communication pathways remaining to us.

Reading through my sometimes-bare journal entries from those times brings them back to life for me, and I find myself filling in the gaps from my memory.

Saturday, March 17, 2012 [one year after Clair entered KCC].
Clair smiles with delight and, I think, surprise on greeting me.
Putting my arm around her after a good hug and walking back

to her room, as we both laugh, I ask, "You were expecting Clark Gable?" More laughter.

As we stroll to the isolated trail across the street from KCC, we negotiate a marsh of muck and water, the result of recent wind and rainstorms. She follows me bravely through the safest portion of the slough, holding my hand, then points out dry patches along the other side of our trail where "we don't have to step on turds!" I pick up the beat near the end of our outdoor hike with an extemporaneous poem:

> As we watch the birds . . .
> And avoiding those turds,
> I have only some words,
> Of Beauty . . . for you: I love you!

Clair smiles warmly yet remains silent. On the way in, I hack up a sputum, and after I spit on the ground, she scolds me, "Don't do that, please!" (She is still Clair.) But an attempt to respond to her comment, maybe to discuss it, goes nowhere.

Inside KCC we march pretty much directly to her room where I help remove her sweater and weather breaker. I take off her shoes and mine, and together we lie on her single bed, holding each other. I make up a simple poem and tell her, "I love you, Clair! . . . and I am yours!"

"Me too!" she echoes, her eyes softly closed beneath her glasses, a contented, gentle smile on her face.

As I continue to kiss her on her forehead, cheek and cheekbone, she caresses my forearm. We are together, close, warm, safe, both loving and loved. *This* is mutuality, David! I silently remind myself. Being on one—or more—of the same pages with Clair at the same time. Shared history. Feeling close to each other, hearing each other with neither contradiction nor criticism, but fully. Being there *with* each other. And inwardly I remind myself, Now stop complaining that you don't experience mutuality with your wife anymore, okay? I smile at my own nearsightedness and sag back onto her bed, both happy and content.

I help put her shoes on again, and then still on my knees I promise her, "One more kiss. You decide where you want it!" She leans over and gently, warmly, sensuously kisses me tenderly full on my lips. It is a long, slow, loving, wet kiss.

I lapse comfortably back into my memory bank of the over 5,000 nights we have snuggled, cuddled, nuzzled and snoozled each other. And I know if I wait—or don't wait, but hesitate, falling farther and more contentedly into her warm body and skin—that I will indeed fall asleep in her arms for the night. In our duet of heat and warmth, warmth prevails by one quarter note.

On my way out, just as I near the door, she calls "David!" Already feeling gifted, I turn to her for another embrace. This is the first time she has called me David in maybe five or six months!

Walking to the bus stop, I am about six inches off the ground, and I hear myself begin to sing "Hava Nagila," the Hebrew folk song that says, "Let us rejoice and be glad!" The words are almost, though not quite, singing themselves. I am the voice box that the lyrics are springing from and a happy, contented member of the audience at the same time!

That night at about eight o'clock the very competent charge nurse at KCC phoned to say, "I wanted you to know that Clair has had a fall. We found her sort of sitting on the floor in the hallway!" A pair of bookends, I thought. Possibly the closest Clair and I would ever be again followed just six hours later by a thump! [What I didn't realize then was that this was a sign of Clair's new difficulty in walking, the beginning of the ataxic gait that would see her in a wheelchair within two years.]

After I put the phone down, I found myself thinking about some of the questions to which I was just beginning to find answers. First, how do you love someone who is disappearing right in front of your eyes? You already love your partner, and you are not changing—or at least not changing as quickly as your partner is. Your challenge *and* opportunity is to continue being yourself while still loving your partner as you did yesterday. But you must be careful about confusing love with sexuality, with intimacy, maybe even with tenderness. These wonderful experiences all overlap with each other, entwining and complementing each other, yet they can—and must of necessity—be disentangled and experienced separately as your partner's AD or other dementia progresses.

What I was learning, and what Clair was teaching me, was that we could *bypass* sex in the journey to lovemaking. I had wanted both sexual warmth and heat from Clair, but she had—and continued to remind me that she had—either forgotten about sex or no longer had an interest in it, or both. However, she still seemed to need, want and appreciate warmth as much as I did. This situation called for some resilience from me, her partner, as we nonverbally renegotiated, reconsidered old pathways of connection and experimented with and practised learning new ones. How to do that? I was trying to do it in a way that seemed and felt comfortable to both of us, improvising and using my ingenuity. On a good day I managed to be brave and bold, but also as kind and thoughtful as I could manage to be.

Second, I had learned that when your partner no longer calls you by your name or pet name, it does *not* mean that you are no longer the most important person in his/her life. So let me caution you *not* to personalize your partner's continuing memory defects and the manner in which they spill over into language. Do not correct them, *and do not argue with them*. I would still remind Clair at times that my name was David, and she would tolerate this with good humour, but I did it more for fun and for my own peace of mind and well-being than in the hope that she would be likely to remember the next time. (It is worth noting that the last time she used my name was *not* the last time we snuggled so warmly together.)

Third—and forgive me for reminding you what you already know— I had learned that both sexuality and tender intimacy occur within the moment, the here and now. Enjoy the closeness you might be feeling with your partner and savour it. Do you want to push your luck and go for a sexual connection after that? Sure, but don't push too far, and don't forget to listen to and look for cues and clues from your beloved. And don't—*do not*—look a gift horse in the mouth. Enjoy what—and who—is in front of you and what is between you, the richness, the possible intensity, the full- ness and the vibrancy of that time you are sharing with each other. Enjoy the moment—or be frustrated, even left longing—today, and still look forward to this evening or tomorrow with your partner. A little frustra- tion, fear and anxiety can follow a disappointing moment that may follow a fantasy or two of expectation, but give yourself some wiggle room to look forward to a close time with your partner again soon.

> **Monday evening, May 14, 2012.** A marvellous time with Clair this afternoon. She welcomed me warmly, and after hugging me, she noted, "You've just had a haircut!" She is still the perceptive psychologist and the person I remember so fondly. Out we went for a walk in the most beautiful, sunny BC weather we've enjoyed in some time. Coming to the first fork in our pathway through the conifer and deciduous woods, I offered her a choice, she opted for the longer route, and we continued our walk, hand in hand. Once or twice I stopped and hugged her, and she responded warmly. We enjoyed long and tender kisses.
>
> I teased her, singing campfire songs to her, and she smiled in apparent enjoyment. I made up a few verses that had her name in the rhyme. She laughed. I was so delighted that her sense of humour was with us today! Then it hit me again: this was that mutuality I had been complaining about missing all this

time. So stop thinking about it, I told myself, and just enjoy it in whatever form or fashion it is available! Both of us seem to be alive, connected and attached *only* in this moment. And what else is there?

Several German shepherd-cross dogs approached us from behind, one of them jumping on Clair with muddy paws, its apologetic owner soon arriving to rescue us. Clair brushed the dog's muddy prints off silently, easily and with grace. I also swatted off some mud, and we continued our jaunt. Heading back to KCC, she wondered out loud if we were "going to our place?" I confirmed this, appreciating her generally sharp state of mind. If Alzheimer's is an ongoing one-step-forward, two-steps-back process, this was definitely one of those one-step-forward days. Or was it just that Clair and I had found each other again in the moment? I felt close to her and told her so, singing another made-up song celebrating our love. She smiled.

Sunday, June 10, 2012. I walked all the way to visit Clair early this afternoon, quite a trek, but I felt good, if tired, when I finally arrived at KCC. I sat down beside my sweetie, and she seemed pleasantly surprised to see me, then continued watching *I Love Lucy* with her friend Harry [not his real name] sitting on her right side. He seemed to be half asleep. It was five or six minutes before I noticed that their hands were clasped.

"We're just holding hands!" the now more awake Harry assured me.

"That's fine!" I reassured him, taking Clair's left hand and making a small joke about her having two beaus now. Neither of them laughed at my feeble humour, though Clair responded warmly, if passively. I kissed her on her left cheek, telling her how much I loved her. She smiled.

She and Harry were still holding hands, though he was now slumped, again about half asleep. Then gently Clair removed her left hand from mine. I reached for her hand again, and she neither resisted nor responded warmly to this gesture, but her right hand and Harry's left one continued in gentle contact. I silently reminded myself, David, you knew there was a strong possibility that this step could be coming!

I wanted to take Clair back to her room and do some of the old-fashioned snuggling that we had enjoyed so many times, but that didn't feel quite appropriate. You're on a sort of double date here,

David, I silently told myself. On my way out, I walked behind Clair's
chair and kissed her goodbye on the top of her head, as was often
my custom. She and a sleepy Harry were still holding hands.

That occasion would be the only time I would see Clair and Harry
together, yet it was a big event for me, and the memory is still etched
somewhere within the anxious part of my cerebral cortex. I remembered
reading that the husband of retired US Supreme Court Justice Sandra
Day O'Connor had found companionship with a woman resident in the
nursing home in which he lived. They reportedly spent most of their time
together, holding hands even in the presence of Justice O'Connor. Her son
Scott told a reporter for *USA Today* that this development was a relief to his
mother and that she was pleased that his father was relaxed and happy.[6] I
also took comfort in the words of Tara Parker Pope of the *New York Times*
who, when commenting on this situation, noted that doctors say it is not
unusual for people with AD to seek out new partners within their care
community.[7] The memories may go slowly or quickly, but the need for
friendship, companionship and love often continue for some time. Justice
O'Connor's reaction to her husband's new friendship, together with her
gracious, selfless behaviour, was palpably helpful and comforting. So even
as I sat next to Clair, nestled there between Harry and me, I felt a mixture
of relief, curiosity and sadness, together with an appreciation and gratitude
for the moment, for the two of them and their experience.

So how do we negotiate the frequently changing boundaries with our
AD partners—for example, when he/she develops a crush or maybe even
a deeper affection for another person in his/her care residence? What did
I learn from this turn of events? First, that I would get over it. As will you,
but don't expect not to have feelings, possibly—even probably—conflicts
over your AD partner's need for new friends and maybe for affection and
physical comfort as well. She/he is not exchanging you for someone new.
Your partner is in a new world, starting over. You may still be part of his/
her life, but like all friendships and partnerships, your relationship will
not be as it was five or ten or fifteen years ago. Now the changes are, and
will continue to be, more dramatic, challenging and at times subjectively
overwhelming. Honour your feelings about these changes, and do not keep
them to yourself. Share them with a friend or two, a trusted family member, a counsellor or all three. Write about it, as I have. Pray on it, if that is
comforting to you, or meditate, or both. This will be a rich learning experience for you.

Monday, July 23, 2012. I had not seen Clair for ten days as I had
been visiting my children and grandchildren in southern Oregon.

I missed her more than I had appreciated, and we scurried pretty much straight to her room after I arrived. I was not tuning into any mixed feelings on her part or mine as I just wanted to be with her, to be close to her. Physically? Emotionally? My heart, mind, body and soul were not caught up with that distinction. "Everywhere, every way possible!" they cried in unison. I told myself, Stop splitting hairs, David, and just let yourself go. Clair's not resisting, is she?

Along with tenderness I also felt sexual passion that day— warmth interwoven with heat—and without thinking I placed her hand on top of my bulging trousers, where she caressed me gently, if briefly. Then I spontaneously took her hand and started to pull it down under my pants and underpants to my genitals.

Without missing a beat, she grabbed my right thumb and, while laughing, crowed, "I've got it!" We both immediately laughed at her fast comeback. She was *still* Clair. Then I gently and silently scolded myself: David, let it go! Time's up for that! And *she's* been pretty much consistent with her receptivity, or lack of it, over the last months, eh? The problem is that you're *still David*—you horny bastard!

Later as I walked to the bus stop, I experienced a sharper sense of exactly who Clair and I were now and, lubricated by a shared sense of humour, were perhaps becoming. As long as at least one of us is laughing and having fun, I told myself, we are moving along the right pathway. And if both of us are laughing, then we have the secret!

Friday, July 27, 2012. Again Clair seemed happily surprised to see me, and I joined her at her dinner table. She was slow to feed herself that day, and I fed her the better part of her meal—but as we neared the end of it and a delicious berry cobbler arrived, she took the initiative and fed herself more. My observing ego stepped away from us, whispering in my ear, "David, you've not been this solicitous with Clair previously. Feeding her forkful by forkful! What's going on here, anyway?"

Of course, I knew what was happening, but I had a problem acknowledging it at the time. This was a precursor of things to come. We had been going from wife and husband to friend and friend, and now we were moving to a more caretaking and supportive, nurturing arrangement. Clair and

I were separately and together moving another step along the caretaking/ caregiving/care-receiving continuum—as you will be doing if you have not already moved forward to that point. You don't have to like it—but you also don't have to fight it. Relax and accept the inevitability of it. And with a little practice, and maybe a few potholes in your shared journey along the AD road, both you and your partner will adapt and adjust.

Staying with your loved one during changes and transitions in your partnership will also see you staying with your memories of who you were, apart and together, before AD visited your lives. Try not to tune out or disappear physically, emotionally or psychologically in this process. By staying with those memories and staying with your partner today, you *honour* the memories of what you shared and enjoyed together yesterday and what you experience together today. In so doing, you give your partnership, your marriage, your relationship the continuity that will see you through to tomorrow.

With these thoughts tumbling through my head, I invited Clair to join me in her room, and she agreed, taking my hand as we walked. In her room I couldn't help but chuckle at the large hand-written sign resting atop a pair of her slacks. During a walk earlier in the week I had noticed they were much too long for her, and now in letters more than three-quarters of an inch high, one of the staff had written: HUSBAND WILL HEM.

After I invited Clair to join me in bed, I took off my shoes, then hers, and she laughed when I kissed her toes through her not-recently-laundered socks. When I lay down on the right side of her bed, I noticed she was still sitting on the left, her legs over the side. Not until after I encouraged her to swing her legs up alongside mine did I remember that she had been assuming this sitting position the last six or seven times when I invited her to snuggle—a possible signal of a new reticence or mixed feelings that I had overlooked until today. Being more careful than usual, I lay down to spoon with her, and she gently stroked my hands and right forearm with her left hand. I observed out loud, "Sometimes people may not want to do this . . . and they can say yes . . . no . . . maybe . . . or even 'I'm not sure right now.'"

She was quiet, neither withdrawing from nor approaching me more closely, but she grimaced, and for a moment I thought she was about to cry. No tears came. She mumbled several words but could not or would not repeat them for me. Then I asked her outright, "Would you like to snuggle, honey? Or is that maybe about enough for now?"

She paused before she answered simply, "That's a good question!" She was quiet again, her eyes mostly closed.

Slowly I collected my things, put on my loafers and let myself out. On my way to my bus stop holding the bag containing her slacks, I experienced a mixture of relief, sadness and grief. Had I read her signals accurately? Or were these signals I had previously overlooked? Or was it mostly my eagerness to get some answers—any answers—that would help me to at least begin to write an ending for this newest chapter of our marriage, which I wanted so badly to write, within this desert of grief, anxiety, quiet ambiguity, uncertainty and heartbreak?

|||||||||||||||||||||||||||||||||

My intimate relationship with Clair would diminish persistently across the later months of 2012 and through the following year, although it was not until I looked back over the entries in my journal that I recognized the progressions and regressions. There were visits that were warmly rewarding, but there were others when I had to acknowledge sudden, sharp downturns and losses in our relationship. One or more features of who we were previously would be missing, whether in emotional, psychological, physical, comforting or intimate ways or in some combination of them. We were slowly edging onto a starvation diet. If you are consuming 2,000 calories a day this week, then eat 1,900 calories a day next week, you might not appreciate the difference. But what about the third week, when you restrict yourself to 1,800 calories a day? Or the fourth week? I have selected a few of the visits during this period to demonstrate those one-step-forward, two-steps back days, so difficult for me to appreciate or articulate when I was in the midst of them.

> **Sunday, October 7, 2012.** Clair welcomed me with a look of pleased surprise together with a cautious embrace on my arrival at KCC this morning.
>
> I asked her, "What do you think, honey? A walk? Snuggle? Maybe a nice talk?"
>
> "Maybe fifty-fifty!" she suggested, and with that I took her hand and we walked to her room, to our room. As I opened the door, she seemed curious that I had a key, but I could not decipher anything else she shared in her whispered fragments of speech. The bed alarm went off several times, and I quieted it while softly cursing. I took off my runners, but when I suggested that I take off Clair's shoes, she resisted, though she sat down on her side of the bed.
>
> Okay, I thought as I sat beside her, this is a new chapter perhaps. "I'm guessing, Clair," I wondered out loud, "that you don't want to say no to snuggling, but maybe you don't want to say yes either. Is that sort of it?"
>
> She nodded just a bit and murmured, "Yeah!"

And with that, I lay down on my side of her bed as usual. After a moment or two she lay down next to me, flat on her back with her head nestled on my left shoulder. I began softly kissing her right cheek and forehead, and telling her right from my heart that I loved her. This felt so good and Clair seemed so quietly accepting that I turned over to face her, attempting to nudge my right leg between her legs, but she kept her position, with her legs crossed at the ankles. I sang a crude allegory spontaneously in no particular key, "I'm just a little orphan leg with no place to call home! Maybe I should knock on the door for somebody to let me in!"

Clair neither laughed nor smiled. I caressed her sweatered arm, and she gently and softly stroked my hand. Her shoes were still on as we lay together, her legs still crossed at her ankles.

After twenty minutes or so, I kissed her once more, reminding her, "I'll see you soon, love!" As I headed for her door after collecting my things, I looked back and saw that she had separated her legs ever so slightly, while looking in another direction. And just before I closed her door, I noticed that she had crossed her legs again at the ankles. I was puzzled by my feelings as I headed for the bus. Clair had just given me an open, authentic and sincere gift—eloquent, muscular, honest body language. And this is how I remember her during our first eighteen years together: a strong woman who always put honesty and clarity before hurt feelings or protecting someone else's poise, pride or balance.

Monday, October 22, 2012. Recreation worker Rosabel has invited Clair and me to join in a game of Recognize the Celebrity, in which she held up a photo of a movie star, singer or dancer from the 1950s or '60s and asked us all to guess his/her identity. She is a virtuoso at laughing with us, stopping short of laughing at us, and she asked Clair if she would leave me for Cary Grant. Clair paused before saying softly, "I'm not sure!" provoking a fair amount of laughter, including some from me.

At a stopping point in the game, I took Clair's hand to lead us to her room, but she resisted, stopping to say hello to someone. I returned to my armchair, and she sat down again next to me. The group, which again included Clair and myself, was still involved in the game and it continued with warm, raucous laughter.

Asking her later if she would like to go for a snuggle got no response, and I ceased and desisted, though I persisted in holding and stroking her hands. Our snuggling time was shortening, and I accepted this with a peace of mind that surprised me. As I left, she looked at me briefly, then turned her attention elsewhere.

Looking back on that October day, I realize that I had now accepted the fact that any answers were better than no answers. Is the devil we know better than the devil we don't know? Adrift in uncertainty and grief, I was now comforted with a more visible, palpable shoreline of greater clarity, and I could see it from where I was treading water. It was certainly not the shoreline I had been seeking, yet it *was* a shoreline. And I would now be able to rest while I caught my breath and grieved simultaneously.

You can live comfortably with both uncertainty and ambiguity within your relationship with a loved one suffering from dementia, but a small amount of courage will help. Staying in focus, sharply and clearly within the here and now with your beloved, will become easier with practice and with time. Don't forget to share special moments like these with friends, family or your counsellor. When you do, you will often still be alone, but you are unlikely to feel lonely.

Monday, November 5, 2012. This afternoon I suggested to Clair, "We could go into our room and snuggle . . . if you want." To this she began to respond, "I don't . . .," but her voice trailed off. Our hands continued to hold each other for another ten minutes, but when I became more assertive, inviting her to her room, she agreed. Once there, I invited her to join me on the bed, which she did after letting me remove her shoes, but it seems there would be no more spooning between us as she lay flat on her back close to me. When I asked her what she would like, she responded quickly, "I want to see Robert!" which I acknowledged. My indelicate and impulsive suggestion that I kiss her private parts prompted her quick, sharp response.

"No!" she snapped. Then she added, "Maybe next week!"

There was no ambiguity there, although she seemed quite comfortable lying beside me, both of us on our backs yet close to each other. When I suggested we go to chow, she sat up and proceeded to put on her right shoe and my left one. When I pointed this out, she allowed me to take back my shoe and help her put on her own left shoe. I seated her at the dining table, but she stood up again and tried to follow me out the door.

Wednesday, November 7, 2012. Clair was delighted to see me today, bounding away from Rosabel's occupational therapy group and their painting project.

"Well, what am I, chopped liver?" Rosabel teased.

Clair ignored the good-natured banter and fell right into my arms. I fetched another chair and, after returning Clair's newly repaired glasses to her face, suggested that we sit together for the balance of Rosabel's group, in which they were discussing the athletic exploits of the residents. I reminded the residents and staff that Clair had been the fastest woman in her age group to climb the Grouse Grind six or seven years earlier. Then I reminded Clair of the achievement and told her how proud I was of her. She acknowledged my fond words of praise with vague mumbles that left me wondering how much of this remarkable exploit she actually remembered.

What was I trying to do with this interchange anyway? I'm not sure, but maybe I was trying to share with Rosabel's group the Clair I was so proud of and loved so much. And maybe trying to share Rosabel's group with a withdrawn Clair. Or possibly sharing myself with both Clair *and* her group.

I suggested we go back to Clair's room for a cuddle, and hand in hand we walked to the new room to which she had been moved because of her increasing ataxia, the stumbling gait that accompanied her growing number of falls. This room was closer to the nursing station and would allow the nurses and aides to watch her more closely. After I took off my outdoor gear, she allowed me to remove her shoes. As I lay down as usual on the right side of her bed, she immediately took one of my shoes and laced it up on her right foot, but it was only after she had rearranged our three remaining shoes that she hesitantly lay down on her bed next to me, flat on her back. Looking down at the floor space next to her side of the bed, I noted that she had paired up her right shoe with my left one, the two of them pointing to her window to the outside world. A more eloquent image for our relationship today I could not have imagined.

I asked Clair if she would like to rest her head on my shoulder. "I shortly . . . will," she replied. She then asked, "Lift your leg, please!" I hadn't been aware that either of my legs was in her space but nevertheless rearranged my legs. And we lay there together, Clair on her back, me on my left side next to her, her right hand gently holding my right arm wrapped around her torso, as I tried unsuccessfully for the spooning position I had previously enjoyed so much. My kisses were tender, and I told her how much I loved her.

She did not protest, complain or validate what I had said. Our palpable, shared warmth remained interwoven with my additional heat for another ten or fifteen minutes. After getting up, I asked Clair to tell me about her left shoe and my right shoe, so close together. She mumbled something I did not understand. We walked out to her place at her dining table where I fastened her bib in place and kissed her goodbye. As I moved to the exit, I noticed her glancing at me ever so briefly, but she then turned her gaze to her dining partner. My thoughts and feelings were a bit jumbled as I left KCC. I felt more distant from her, yet full of a different sort of love for her than I can ever remember experiencing.

What was this new fondness? As I sorted it out, it seemed to be partly a father's tender love for his daughter. A boy's deep love for a favourite cousin, bringing back memories of my childhood. Perhaps like loving a pet? No, that was damning with faint praise. But how to express the inexpressible? And what must it be like for Clair, with confused feelings for a loved one who is now becoming more like a guest, a stranger she often still enjoys, though possibly with diminishing trust.

February 8, 2013. It's about 5:15 on a Friday evening in February, and I have just left Clair wrapped in her bib in preparation for her dinner at KCC. I'm standing at the bus stop as the home-going traffic whizzes up and down Mount Seymour Parkway. A beautiful, almost full moon hangs between two conifers, lighting up the southeastern sky over the Lower Mainland. A watery liquid drains slowly out of my eyes. This can't be tears, can it? I'm not sad or anything like that, am I? And why should I be sad, anyway? I dismiss it as a reaction to the evening's cold weather.

An hour earlier, after being warmly greeted by Clair, I quickly scooped her up, escorted her back to her room, unlocked her door, let us both in and gently deposited her on her usual side of the bed. After dumping my outer winter clothing and taking off my shoes, I returned to Clair's feet. First, off came her shoes. Then wanting to be closer to her, I took off both her socks. Then I asked her to pick a foot for me to serenade. After some hesitation, she pointed to her left foot. "Eeny-meeny-miney-mo!" I sang as I kissed each toe from her big toe to number four. "And this one we'll call your . . . little toe!" She laughed gently, though not out loud, both of us enjoying the affectionate silliness of the moment, I think. I know I was!

Then I switched to her right foot, "Matthew, Mark, Luke, John! And this one [her big toe] we'll all rely upon!" The earthy smell of her toes somehow added to the close immediacy, emotion and fun I was having, flirting and playing with Clair. I left her feet and toes, encouraged her to scoot up higher in the bed, and wrapped my arms around her while we spooned, our bare feet comforting each other. "Your feet are cold!" she scolded me tenderly and was then quiet, her eyes calmly closed as we lay comfortably, contentedly together for the next fifteen or twenty minutes.

We talked more than we had for a while—in other words, a little bit. She would murmur a phrase, and I would try, usually unsuccessfully, to decipher it. "We should look at it," I thought she said, but when I repeated those words, she shook her head. So I repeated or paraphrased her words less often, and she became simultaneously quieter. We were silent again, the medium that had found us so tenderly, quietly close during my visits over the last two or three weeks. I could have lain there for another hour or two, but dinnertime was approaching. After we both stood up, her bed alarm sounded, bringing a nurse to turn it off, almost apologetically. Clair and I walked to her table, and I fastened her bib. I told her I'd see her soon, then let myself out, sending her a goodbye kiss as she looked at me kindly, comfortably, without any discernible longing.

So now I wondered as I stood waiting for my bus, what was this watery substance flowing from my eyes if not tears? Being closer to Clair that quiet afternoon had been both a balm and a reminder of what we had enjoyed earlier in our marriage, only on more levels both broader and deeper—intellectual, social, psychological, even political. What remained, it seemed, was just closeness. So, David, I told myself, you have enjoyed and continue to enjoy gifts with Clair. Don't be ungrateful. Then I reminded myself that I had experienced in this tender afternoon perhaps more closeness with my partner than many married people might enjoy within six months, perhaps even a year or longer.

Thursday, March 14, 2013. I had not seen Clair for over two weeks, first because of a norovirus quarantine at KCC and then because I had been visiting my family in southern Oregon. Within a few seconds of my arrival I spotted her comforting an agitated friend. She smiled briefly on seeing me, but offered no hugs as she had done recently. She welcomed me warmly, but not as her husband or even as a close friend, but as a sort of a friend of a friend—warmly, yet somewhat diffident and unsure of the nature of our relationship. I told her a little about my trip to Oregon and how much I had missed her, then invited her to join me in her room where staff had suggested we meet since the recent quarantine. She walked away from me with words I could not understand. I followed her while trying to allow her some distance from me at the same time. She stayed away from her room, though when I put my key into the lock, she allowed me to invite her in with me. I asked her to join me on her bed, took off her shoes and, seeking tenderness and intimacy with her, kissed her big toe protruding through a hole in her right sock. No response. With some encouragement, she lay down beside me in an L-shaped posture with her lower trunk and legs pointed away from me at ninety degrees. But as I held her, ever so tentatively she softly stroked my right arm.

After I reminded her that she could refuse to snuggle with me and that I would honour her wishes, she said quickly with a slight laugh, "You'd better!" *Still* Clair. I sang to her, rubbed her back and stroked the smooth-as-silk skin on her warm hands and arms, but she continued her L-shaped posture. When I invited her to join me more closely, she responded with something that sounded like "No, thank you," or "Not now."

She seemed more emotionally distant from me than ever I remembered . . . and when I pointed to a sixteen-year-old photo of me on her chest of drawers and asked if she knew that man, she replied simply, "I used to." I could not have said it better. Before I let myself out, she murmured some words that sounded like "I can't feel anyone." Attempts to get her to repeat this were followed by silence. She did allow me to kiss her several times, warmly and tenderly but briefly, like a small girl might allow her Daddy to kiss her on his return from work. As I left, her eyes were quietly closed. I told her I'd see her soon.

The next day when I recounted this experience to a close friend, he said, "Now that the quarantine is over and you are back in town and begin to visit more often, maybe she will be less of a stranger." My friend was right; Clair did respond more warmly to me on my next visit two days later. One step backward, one step forward, I reminded myself with relief. But better not keep score, David. Better to enjoy each other as long as you can, where you are, where she is and in the moment. I was finally beginning to grasp what I had previously dismissed as a cliché—the *here and now*—and to understand the mindfulness and sharper sense of attention that allow us, encourage us, to fully appreciate and enjoy it. What I had forgotten almost since the time of Clair's diagnosis and in my continuing search for closeness and sexual and nonsexual intimacy was that *without* that closeness and without that partner that Clair once was—and also without that evanescent partner I continued to search for—I, David, was *also* still a person. I was still someone. I had not disappeared—well, not that much, anyway— just because Clair continued to leave me, her friends, her family and her world one teaspoon at a time.

> **Monday, May 26, 2013.** Bus to KCC for a lovely, warm nap and snuggle with my Clair. I had learned a lot in the two and one-half years that she'd been in care—about her, about me, about us and the intimacy we have shared and grown into and that I continued to seek under new and challenging circumstances. And I wondered—what have those two and one-half years been like for her? What has she learned?

During the late spring and early summer of 2013 I continued to visit Clair about every two days, almost sure I would not experience that special closeness and tenderness that she and I had enjoyed on that May 26 visit. I was wrong. After watching her physically and sexually slipping away from me for more than eighteen months, I logged the following note in my journal:

> **Saturday, June 1, 2013.** Another lovely snuggle with Clair—that's twice in three visits!

What I remember about that particular visit but did not log in my journal at the time was the immense closeness and tenderness I experienced with her. She seemed mentally sharp that day, and as we ended a walk in the woods, I told her mushy things like I'd "like to kiss you all over. Love you forever. To eternity. Surrender to you. Take care of you and protect you." To which she responded dryly, "I think I could handle that!"

Later, as we lay side-by-side on her bed, her legs relaxed, she allowed me to spoon more closely with her in a manner I'd not—or we'd not—enjoyed in probably a year. When she rolled over onto her back and put her head on my shoulder, I kissed her tenderly on her forehead and cheeks. Her hands caressed me tenderly and wandered near my erection. On an impulse I placed her hand there. She neither caressed me—no surprise—nor withdrew her hand, and I experienced much pleasant and tender amazement.

I surrendered to Clair's warmth in the moment, savouring it, wondering if she was perhaps also experiencing similar feelings. I was grateful and happy.

I remember walking to my bus that day in deep, quiet gratitude, once again reminding myself not to base my predictions for today on what I, or we, had experienced yesterday. Probably the most essential thing I had learned in all this time was the importance of listening to Clair with my mind, my heart, my body and my soul, a concept I was just now really understanding. I had learned to love her with and without words, with and without touch, with and without plans, birthdays, anniversaries, parties or expectations. I had learned the importance of friends and faith. I now prayed less for myself while praying thanks and gratitude more—though I was not sure if I was praying to God or just saying thanks.

|||||||||||||||||||||||||||||||||

So what can you as a caregiver of a partner with Alzheimer's learn, what would you *like* to learn, about sexuality and intimacy from my experience with Clair over these months and years while she was at home and then in care?

First, you need to become more comfortable with the physical, intimate and sexual parameters and varied aspects of your relationship even as—*especially* as—the windows into your partnership begin to fog up and narrow. I think Clair moving away from me physically in our made-for-snuggling bed at KCC could not have been more of an honest statement of our changing relationship. In retrospect, I understood that we were indeed leaving each other and that the on-again off-again but inexorably widening distance was an undeniable message from her. So a first big step for me was the recognition of this message, accepting that it was time to redefine the loving experience while searching for a new and different sort of closeness. For me, however, and probably for you, fully understanding and appreciating the width and depth and breadth of that new kind of closeness might take a while longer.

Second, do not be surprised if at times, as your partner is disappearing from you, you feel as though you may love him or her more. Even if this does not happen, you may expect to appreciate more than ever the love that you have shared, your partnership with all its ups and downs and the memories you continue to experience. That appreciation has been an enormous gift for me, and it can or will be a gift for you as well. Kahlil Gibran reminded us of this gift when he wrote: "Love knows not its own depth/ Until the hour of separation." The gift that keeps on giving—appreciation of my love of and for Clair and of the partnership we shared—is today bordered by a wider and deeper appreciation of the human condition, of people and all their gifts.

Third, and perhaps most important, you will need to take care of yourself, your own level of sexual need, desire, fantasy and frustration, your need for companionship, for social friendship, contact and support. If spiritual or religious needs are important to you, by all means value and respect them, respond to them, nurture them, and at times give yourself a break and let them run some of your show. I urge you to be true to yourself and the parts that help make up that self in a manner and on a timetable that you are comfortable with and that is also consistent with your own morality and belief systems; and remember that by being true to yourself, you honour your partner and what you have shared and enjoyed, together and apart, over the years of your relationship.

Some of what I have shared here about consent and permission, the distinctions between them and the overlap of warmth and heat between two individuals may reflect your own situation. Some may seem totally irrelevant or extraneous to your relationship with your AD partner. And perhaps much will fall in between these two extremes. Although I don't have an exact blueprint or a map for where you could or should go in the changing nature of the sexuality and intimacy you share with your loved one, I am strongly committed to the vision that with patience, curiosity and loving kindness, you will find your own pathways to follow through each of these experiences—lovemaking, love, sex, kindness, tenderness, intimacy and closeness together and apart from your partner. They will be different experiences, yet they will often overlap in unpredictable ways.

Follow your intuition as you look back on your lives together and apart, and above all, listen to your instincts and intuition and feelings as you seek to keep in touch with your partner. What did the two of you enjoy and appreciate in the days before her/his AD? What do you still find comforting and warming now? What do you experience that keeps you close to each other today, or brings you even closer? The answers to these important questions of intimacy and sexuality will help guide the two of you in the months and years to come in your new living environment.

|||||||||||||||||||||||||||||||||

Finally, we must talk about one of the peculiarities of dementia: that it can cause those affected to either be less like themselves, even more like themselves or unexpectedly *both*. This means that you should always expect the best possible connections with your loved one while at the same time being ready for other outcomes. Women sometimes find themselves faced with a somewhat unpleasant scenario when it comes to intimacy with an AD spouse. It may still be possible for them to enjoy close physical warmth and contact or pleasing verbal and nonverbal exchanges, but dementia can often be disinhibiting, and a male AD partner may become rough and physically aggressive, or even try to assault or rape. (On the other hand, it is worth knowing that erectile dysfunction is estimated to hover around the 50 percent mark in men with Alzheimer's.[8]) If that AD partner has a previous history of physical or sexual abuse, there is even more reason to be cautious. If unsure, women should always have a chaperone nearby when sharing time and space with their AD partners. If a woman's AD partner is *also* a woman, there may be less reason for caution, yet the suggestions above still apply.

Men, do not be put off by your AD partner's possible reticence in lovemaking. Instead, be patient. Be creative. Be kind. She is a different person from the one you married or committed to, but she is also still your loved one. But do *not* take advantage of your partner's vulnerabilities. Although she may not say no, that doesn't mean she is saying yes to you. Rape by any other name or rationalization is still a felony crime in North America. And it is *wrong*. There are probably many more men who abuse their partners with AD than there are women who do the same. If you find yourself doing this, **stop**. Get help. If necessary, ask for a chaperone or escort when you are visiting her. If she is still at home, it is all the more reason to follow the above rules. And for men whose partners are also men? All the above cautions apply, but if the AD partner is strong and pushy with a history of assault, rape or other felony, be extra cautious. These previous nefarious parts of his history may surface unexpectedly as his dementia progresses.

Above all, for both women and men caregivers, the rule is, be kind to your partner. Honour your own need for physical and emotional closeness, and take care of yourself in as many ways as possible. Depending on the care circumstances, privacy may or may not be a problem, but even in a care centre you still deserve privacy with your loved one. Make sure you get it, but follow your intuition on whether you want a companion with you for some of your visits.

CHAPTER EIGHT

Into the Future

It was a busy
morning, when about 8:30 a
gentleman in his 80s arrived to have
stitches removed from his thumb.
He said he was in a hurry as he had
an appointment at 9:00 am.
I took his vital
signs and had him take a seat,
knowing it would be over an hour
before someone
would be able to see him.
I saw him looking at his watch and
decided, since I
was not busy with another patient,
I would evaluate his wound.
On exam I saw it was
well-healed, so I talked to one of the
doctors, got the needed supplies to
remove his sutures and redress his wound.

While taking care of
his wound, I asked if he

*had another doctor's appointment
this morning as
he was in such a hurry.*

*The gentleman told me no, that he
needed to go to
the nursing home to eat breakfast
with his wife. I inquired as to her
health.*

*He told me that she had been there
for a while and that she
was a victim of Alzheimer's Disease. I asked if she would be
upset if he was a bit late.*

*He
replied that she no longer knew
who he was, that she had not
recognized him in
five years now.*

*I was surprised and asked,
"And you still go every morning, even though she
doesn't know who are you are?"*

*He smiled as he
patted my hand and said,
"She doesn't
know me, but I still know who she is."*

—Anonymous

This peaceful and serene story-poem, with its snapshot of apparently dogged and unchanging devotion, shows us a man committed to a woman who is no longer even the essence of who she was, yet he is still faithful to the partnership they shared. What we don't know is how difficult it was for him to remain faithful. Did he ever dream of or look for a new love in the years after his wife's diagnosis?

The inner and outer turmoil that men and women in western culture experience when Alzheimer's visits a partnership was highlighted by the controversy that erupted in September 2011 over the Reverend Pat Robertson's comments on Alzheimer's and divorce. During the question-and-answer portion of the regular broadcast of the *700 Club* on the Christian Broadcasting Network, Robertson was asked what advice the caller should give a friend who had begun seeing another woman after his wife had become incapacitated by Alzheimer's disease.

Robertson responded, "I know it sounds cruel, but if he's going to do something, he should divorce her and start all over again, but make sure she has custodial care and somebody looking after her." He added that he wouldn't "put a guilt trip" on anyone who divorces a spouse who suffers from an incurable illness, "but get some ethicist besides me to give you an answer."

Terry Meeuwsen, Robertson's co-host on the broadcast, pointed out that the couple's marriage vows obliged them to take care of each other for better or for worse and in sickness and in health.

"If you respect that vow, you say 'til death do us part," Robertson replied, "but this is a kind of death."

This exchange caused outrage throughout Christian communities and made headlines across North America, but the issue Robertson helped bring out into the open is one that our culture and society would generally rather tiptoe around than discuss or embrace directly. Most people with an AD partner, however, want to face these conflicts more straightforwardly. For most of us, the relationship we build step by step with our partners after the diagnosis of dementia is difficult and challenging, a tale written in several chapters. In my case the first chapter was business as usual. When Clair was diagnosed in 2007, she was still living at home, under-functioning but manageably so. Despite her increasing frustration and irritability with me, we continued to enjoy our time together, especially weekends at our house in Halfmoon Bay, where I would bring her morning coffee in bed and she and I would read the newspapers and the *New Yorker*. These memories are very special, even comforting, and they persist to this day.

In the second chapter a certain amount of anticipatory grieving became part of my day. Sure, AD was progressive, but I had told myself it would be a slow process in our case. Clair's outbursts of unexplained anger, however, reminded me that she was indeed changing. A small part of me was sad, another part anxious, and the really bad days would see me feeling either numb or sorry for myself—or both. Sometimes we would share fantasies of our future in brief conversations, sandwiched in between more enjoyable, more exciting things to do, more current issues and schedules. The future would arrive soon enough. Why talk about it now?

In the third chapter I was compelled to assume the role of caretaker as she fumbled meals in our kitchen (e.g., trying to bake a frozen pizza in our microwave). That role grew as she gradually became too confused to continue work at the clinic and grew even more when she began phoning 911 to report a stranger in our home. Earlier I had been able to comfort her when we cuddled at night, but not in this chapter of our story. Some of her more violent outbursts ended in visits to our neighbourhood hospital, one visit prompted by a probable transient ischemic attack (TIA, or small stroke). Each time the doctors would commiserate, pat her on the back (or so it seemed), write her a sedative prescription and send us home.

One of the cruel ironies in the experience of loss is that new grief often brings up old grief. In the fourth chapter I would find myself missing Betsy, my previous wife, more than ever and would talk to her *in absentia*. Some days I would weep over my Betsy, though less often over Clair, perhaps because in many ways Clair was still right there with me; but occasionally I would find myself crying over both partners at the same time. Only on rare occasions would I share my longings for the old days with Clair, but I frequently reminded her how much she meant to me, *had* meant to me, and how much I dearly loved her. On my best days I would happily scold myself: "David, look at it this way: you've had two wonderful women in your life—almost fifteen years with each! Do you want to light a candle or curse the darkness?" The question usually answered itself.

In the fifth chapter of our story, Clair moved into care and the process of distancing began in earnest. One afternoon in June 2012, while riding home on the bus after a visit with her, I mused on the loss of mutuality in our relationship. It had been a marker of where we were and how far we had travelled on so many levels of our relationship since we had first met eighteen years earlier. But it had begun to disappear even before 2007 when she was diagnosed. Now I began fantasizing what it would be like to experience mutuality with someone again, though with whom I had no idea. At the same time, I knew that whatever Clair and I enjoyed with each other was unique and irreplaceable. The idea haunted me nevertheless, reminding me of both past and future.

I resisted the temptation to look for a new partner, however. It was not that I didn't frequently fantasize about the possibility, but I didn't act on my fantasies, thus giving me more energy to focus on Clair's situation, and my own, as they continued to change, often in unpredictable ways. Meanwhile, as a natural socializer, I began seeing more people for short periods. Going out with (mostly) male friends allowed me to talk and to listen to someone who was on the same or a similar cognitive page, though I still found myself wanting what I'd had with Clair: a partner who would talk and listen closely to me during our days together, and cuddle and sleep with me at night after making wonderful, intimate, consensual love.

Looking back through my journal today, I spotted an entry from that fifth chapter of my life with Clair, one that perfectly exemplified my thoughts at the time.

Sunday, March 4, 2012. Alone by myself most of today, I have been touched by a warm and tender note from a college girlfriend whom I've not seen in fifty years. Since reading it, the words of the chorus from another Beatles song ["With a Little Help From My Friends"] have been drifting through my head, in and out, on and off, throughout the day. Yes, I definitely want someone to love, I told myself. And then a different conversation started in my head.

FIRST DAVID: But, David, you *have* somebody to love—Clair!

SECOND DAVID: Well, yes, I know, but she's not Clair anymore. Her essence is gone.

FIRST DAVID: Sure, we all know that. But you still love her, don't you?

SECOND DAVID: Well, sure, but . . . uh . . . it's not like before . . . five years ago, say.

FIRST DAVID: Of course! But remember, *no marriage* is like it was five years ago! Or even five days ago!

SECOND DAVID: I miss our passion. The heat between us, you know!

FIRST DAVID: You're always talking about her warmth—isn't that enough?

SECOND DAVID: Yes. No. Maybe. I'm so conflicted!

So how do we deal with our impulses or temptations to respond to our fantasies of reaching out to, maybe even connecting with, another person, one who is *not* struggling with dementia? Many of us in this situation will continue the search for intimacy based on our past experience of rewarding, tender, cherished, warm and intimate moments, but the search is inescapably interwoven with our current situation regarding our partner's health, needs and ability to connect with us in meaningful moments. As we face those same issues together as well as separately, at times our needs will overlap with those of our partner and at other times they will vary greatly.

Meanwhile, the business of living alone, getting used to loneliness and the sexual frustration that often accompanies it, is a learning experience. After Clair went into care, I had bounced back and forth between aloneness and loneliness, and often I couldn't tell where one started and the other stopped because most of the time they overlapped. Whenever I was caught in this uncertain space—though it often took a while to realize I was adrift there—I learned to take eight or ten slow, deep breaths, then count slowly while meditating. This practice seemed to bring me back into focus, out of loneliness and back into a sharper sense of where I *had* been—alone but not lonely. And my own therapist would remind me to heed what I often tell my patients—that loneliness is usually just aloneness poorly tolerated.

In the sixth chapter of our Alzheimer's adventure, I became convinced I was ready for a new, sexually and emotionally rewarding relationship, and I began dating a warm, if anxious, fellow psychiatrist. After she spent the night in my bed while I—as agreed—bedded down on my living room couch, I was awakened by the welcome cry of "Action!" Hastening into my bedroom with gleeful anticipation, I was greeted by the spectacle of my new friend with her legs, ankles and feet enfolded in a giant rubber thong while she ordered, "Traction, David! I need traction for my back! Right now!" All I could think while giving her traction was, "David, you are so close to a relationship—but *so very* far away!" Going out with new friends can be a test of courage at any age, but at my age, dating this special but exacting new friend, I also experienced humiliation—and humour. She was not ready for someone who was *certainly* not ready, but fortunately she had discerned my lack-of-readiness problem more quickly than I did, and we parted without bad feelings.

Men and women differ radically in their approaches to the readiness problem. Women are often more comfortable with caretaking and caregiving roles, while at the same time they may overlook their own spiritual, physical, emotional and sexual needs, including the need for a new partnership (although this is a need that can be expected to wax and wane). Here I am reminded of the old saying that women mourn while men replace. Or, as Gloria Steinem—quoting feminist Irina Dunn—famously said, "A woman without a man is like a fish without a bicycle." Thus the possibilities for potentially unfortunate, even disastrous rebound experiences occur far less often for women than for men. In fact, after the loss of a beloved partner to dementia or death, women reconnect more frequently than men do with other important friends for reality testing and feedback, nurturance, support, love and comfort.

Interestingly, no mention of the possibility of a new partnership was made by any of the women caregivers I interviewed for this book. When asked if she had fantasies of a way forward, Margaret, whose husband Donald had died five months earlier, said that she still felt "a little lost." She continued:

> I don't want to go back to teaching . . . I think I'm retired . . . But I'd like to be useful in some way. I don't want to just *take*. Well, you know, I'm reinventing myself . . . getting in touch with myself or whatever you want to call it.

Both my personal and my professional experience have demonstrated to me that men are more likely to rebound into a new relationship before they fully understand and appreciate their deeper emotional and psychological divisions and elements—and often long before they are ready. Men's work, therefore, is to slow down just a bit and to balance the importance of their present AD partnership with the different qualities that make up their own inner selves today and their needs and fantasies to move on with their lives. For example, I recall once I had been very busy loving Clair during an especially warm and tender visit with her, then found my fantasies unfurling on the bus trip back home, imagining an introduction to a beautiful woman whom I saw on the bus. (I comfort myself that consistency is the hobgoblin of small minds!)

Graham, whose wife had died thirteen months before our interview, told me that he began preparing for his future alone long before her death.

> There comes a time when you're going down the road with your partner with Alzheimer's and you come to a crossroads where you can either go down the same road that she's going down— let your health go, let your diet go—or you can come to the realization that your partner is going down towards death and you don't want to go there. So you have to go a different route, and in order to go that route you have to probably eat better, you have to get proper exercise, you have to keep a positive frame of mind, you have to make hard decisions for her care that you might not really want to make. You have to take a whole different road.

> I had to *decide* that I was either going to have a life after Yvonne or I was not. And if you're not going to have a life after your partner goes, then of course you get caught up in her death and you get sucked into this vortex of grief. It's just a downward spiral. You stop going to the gym, you stop eating properly, you start drinking. There's all kinds of good things that you *don't* do and bad things that you *do* as a result of not having the spirit to carry on and make a new life.

> So, you know, that decision helped me because I then started planning financially for continuing on by myself. I started thinking about what was I going to do with different properties that we owned. I started planning exercise-wise because now I was thinking, "Well, I'm going to carry on after Yvonne, and I'm going to survive after she's gone." So that was probably the defining moment for me. It didn't happen all at once, but, you know, there's the fact that I *decided* that I was going to have a life after Yvonne.

When I asked Graham if he contemplated a new partnership, he told me,

> Well, I have a unique situation. Yvonne's caregiver is still living in the house with me. During the course of her looking after Yvonne we got along really, really well in terms of sharing the household

duties. When Yvonne died, [the caregiver] wanted to go back to school and finish her education, so I said, "Why don't you stay here while you finish school? You can live here free as far as I'm concerned." So she has stayed and it's now been a year.

I commented that this was very generous of him, but he responded,

Not really. I mean, that's what she thinks too, and that's what everybody thinks, but you know, I've got a four-bedroom house, and there's no extra cost for heat or electricity . . . and in exchange she helps clean up the house, and yesterday she worked all day in the garden. So it's got nothing to do with generosity. It's got to do with having somebody there to share, you know? Right now she's working twelve hours a day six days a week so she's not there a lot. But you know, many, many times I come home and she's there, and it's "Hi, how are you?" Somebody to talk to. So that's made a *huge* difference. Of course, it's also created a lot of "yak, yak, yak, yak, yak, yak" among a lot of people. Everybody imagines all kinds of things.

When Graham was silent for a few moments, I prompted, "They're projecting their own needs, fears and fantasies, perhaps?" And Graham replied, laughing,

Oh, everybody's projecting all kinds of stuff. One of my kids says, "Dad, if it works for you, that's great." But I've got one kid who's asking, "Well, what's going on? What's happening?" And I said, "Well, you just tell your wife there's nothing happening, and when there is, I'll let you know." But to answer your question, [the caregiver] has been a big help in terms of me getting past Yvonne, and so, you know, whether the relationship will continue, we'll see.

John, still struggling over whether he can care for his wife, Nancy, at home "to the very end," is just beginning to think ahead. Although Nancy's fear of climbing in and out of a boat means she can no longer visit the family's island cottage, he is unwilling to sell it. He told me,

I've been after the kids to use it more, and I told one son the other day that next year I want him to take it over. I said, "I'll pay the bills, but I want you guys to open it up and use it." I've threatened to sell it, but they're resistant to that because they love the place, but they get so busy and they only get over there for two or three weekends a year. And I really don't want to sell it because if Nancy goes into care and I end up with a new friend, then we can enjoy it together. Going over on my own, I've done that a couple of times and it's not a ton of fun.

Eight years after Michael's wife was diagnosed with Alzheimer's disease, he wrote an article about his emotional quandary.

Sometimes circumstances require a person to virtually re-invent themselves, doing so perhaps consciously for the first time in their lives. This is certainly the case for me. A man in my early seventies, my life has been torn apart by the effects of Alzheimer's, my wife of over forty years—the love of my life—having finally to be moved into a care home. Those who share this predicament—and sadly I believe we are legion—will know the challenges involved. Love for the one afflicted does not decrease, but of course it can no longer be reciprocated in practice. This renders one a virtual single person, attempting to lead as normal a life as possible, but still nurturing the emotional ties of a long and happy marriage. At the same time, it is clear that abandoning one's self to the situation would serve no useful purpose, neither that of the sufferer of this terrible disease nor the one bereft. What to do? Many people who find themselves in this situation turn to family for support. But this may not always be available . . . Hence the need to re-invent one's self. Clearly, I am no longer a twenty-five-year-old bachelor (thank God), but my life situation has many similarities. Much time is spent alone. Friends become supremely important, as does the need for faith . . .

In a close marriage such as ours, though friends are important, the relationship itself satisfies much of the need for the shared experience that friends provide. Suddenly there is a void. This can only be filled by reconnecting—in essence, rebuilding one's personal community. It means cultivating new friends and figuring out how to present one's self as an individual. How is one viewed? How to deal with the possibility that some people may perceive the pursuit of an active social life as a betrayal of the afflicted partner?

My approach is to compartmentalize my life. I am present for my wife and visit her daily, bracing myself for the inevitable decline that accompanies the progress of Alzheimer's disease. When I leave the care home, I busy myself with my work (I am not a retired person, and fortunately what I do permits me to work from home). Along with this goes the pursuit of a social life and the discovery that while the pain doesn't entirely go away, it can be held in abeyance and much joy and satisfaction can be found in the company of others. It is in such circumstances that strong and enduring new friendships can be forged.

Some friends in my circle are attractive single women, which raises, in my case at least, the question of sexual attraction and how to deal with it. As well as being best friends, my wife and I enjoyed a healthy sexual intimacy. That, of course, no longer exists, leaving that part of my life unfulfilled. Sexual appetite is supposed to diminish with age. That doesn't seem to be happening for me—life would be less complicated if it were! On the other hand, facing up to a challenge in any of life's arenas is, I believe, the wellspring of vitality. There is no roadmap here. The only recourse is to conscience and the assertion of the demands of personal survival.

Intrigued by the article Michael had written, I arranged to interview him, six years after his wife's death. He was now living in a new home with a new partner. He explained:

Helen and I bought this house together five or six years ago. I met her when we were attending a seminar called Mind Over Matrix, which was designed to help us see past the conditioning that informs most people's lives—mine anyway. And I met Helen there and was very deeply drawn to her and we soon formed a relationship. This happened when my wife was still alive, in care. And when I think back on that, I ask, "Should I feel guilty about that?" Well, I don't because I made sure that my wife was not adversely affected in any way. I would visit her on a daily basis, often twice a day . . . and every time I would go there, she would be cheerful . . . I would take her for walks around the property in her wheelchair and take her to the waterfront . . .

Meeting Helen was wonderful for me. I couldn't—and still can't—believe my good fortune. And not only that, how understanding everybody was. I mean, in a situation like that it could be construed that I was disloyal, betraying my wife and so on. And I did feel a little uncomfortable living with Helen in the condominium [that I'd shared with my wife]. You know, people are nosy and I was on the council of the condo so I knew a lot of people there . . . I think Helen was uncomfortable with it . . . Well, I know she was, but more uncomfortable with me being uncomfortable. Now we have a new life. It's a new chapter in my life.

As Michael suggests, your life story will continue after Alzheimer's disease invades. What will you include in the next chapters?

|||||||||||||||||||||||||||||||||

The seventh chapter in the Alzheimer's story of Clair and David brought me one of the most valuable experiences in my journey: honestly, openly, sincerely and earnestly falling back in love with her. She was no longer the Clair I had begun courting in 1994, nor the woman I had loved so much and married in 1997. But now I found myself falling in love with the Clair of today, the here and now. I'm not sure but I strongly suspect that this is one of the secrets discovered by the gentleman in the poem that begins this chapter.

By this time, Clair and I were communicating mostly through laughter and music. The snuggling we had both enjoyed since we discontinued sexual lovemaking was now only sporadic. I still told her regularly how much she meant to me, how much I loved her, with punctuation marks of tender kisses. And I told her how much I missed her, which was true on several levels, though I didn't elaborate.

Remarkably, this is the secret for *all* of us in a relationship: love the person you are with today, not the person he/she was yesterday or will be tomorrow. Of course, loving someone with dementia provides more dramatic, more vivid, more remarkable—and also tougher and more challenging—pathways on which to travel, yet the principle is the same. All partnerships are the same, or at least similar, in that *none* of us is with the same person we started out with yesterday or will be with tomorrow. We have to stop mourning over who and what we have lost and love the person who is still here—or the remaining parts or features or bits of the person who is still there. Learning these lessons with and from Clair and meditating more, I found myself enjoying the here and now more. I practised living in the moment, and by studying mindfulness and meditating, I sharpened this sense of being here now. I began practising mindfulness when I was walking, being careful where I put my feet when I stepped up or down a slope. When travelling on the bus, I meditated, focusing on my breathing. Even when brushing my teeth, I tried focusing on the movement of my brush and the sensation my teeth and gums were experiencing (while ignoring the four thirty-second intervals encoded in the electric brush).

|||||||||||||||||||||||||||||||||

By the summer of 2013 the bridges that had connected Clair and me were becoming increasingly fragile. Long walks had become difficult for her, so we walked less often and for shorter distances. I continued to sing to her, but could not feel the connection that music had provided us in the past. She laughed some but neither as frequently or as openly.

> **Tuesday, August 27, 2013.** Meditated on the bus on the way to visit Clair at KCC early this afternoon. Saw her sitting on the couch next to the wide screen TV looking at her hands as she idly twiddled her thumbs and fingers. I sat quietly next to her and offered her a cookie. She looked impassively at me, shaking her head before accepting one-quarter of my cookie. I asked her if she would like to go for a walk or maybe a snuggle, and she gently shook her head.
>
> I took a chance and observed out loud that maybe sometimes she might not remember who I was, to which she nodded briefly without looking at me. I asked her again if maybe she might like to go for a walk, and again she shook her head. Then misinterpreting her drawing circles on the palm of my hand with her forefinger, I began lightly caressing her back. After a short while she told me ever so quietly, "I'd rather you didn't do that." I stopped. Another resident drifted by, and Clair attempted to take her hands, but the other patient softly extricated herself. Then connecting briefly with me, Clair leaned down and gently undid my left shoelace. She didn't seem able to retie it and instead carefully laid the two shoelace ends parallel across the top of my shoe.
>
> Shortly after I began caressing Clair's left arm, she murmured quietly but distinctly to me while gesturing with up-and-down slicing motions of her left arm and hand, "There needs to be...," and then fell silent.
>
> "Some distance here?" I wondered.
>
> She nodded quickly and definitely.
>
> We had connected, understood each other, and at that point the light seemed to go out of our visit. I kissed her briefly on the forehead and hair and told her I'd see her soon. She watched me as I walked out; then her gaze returned to the people and space around her.
>
> Walking through the woods to the bus, I stopped spontaneously next to a tall Douglas fir and hugged it, sobbing quietly without tears.

So now here comes the part I never really wanted to write about: letting Clair go, saying goodbye to her. But how do you say goodbye to someone who's still here in body? And did I really want to do this? It didn't *feel* like something I was ready to do. On the other hand, I *was* missing empathy, support, affinity—in short, the full embodiment of a relationship. I could feel it, taste it. I longed for it, fantasized about it. I wanted that feeling of connecting with Clair on the same or a similar mental and emotional wavelength, quietly or in conversation, with the mutual respect and appreciation we had enjoyed for the many years before Alzheimer's came so rudely into our lives.

So here I was in the middle. I didn't want to say goodbye, but I realized—however painful the realization was—that I was almost ready to move on. Or maybe to take more care of my own needs. The irony here is that I had experienced more closeness, more tenderness with Clair during the last few months than perhaps ever before, though I recognized that this was a different kind of closeness, a closeness without any discernible reciprocity or feedback. At the same time, I had become more alive, more sensitive, alert and receptive in facing the death of our relationship and more sharply focused on my own needs. I wondered quietly why this terrible disease had made it impossible for me to meet my needs with Clair instead of with some other woman or two or three out there within the dating–courtship–mating cycle. However, time—or at least a greater awareness of and sensitivity to its passing—weighs more heavily on my fantasies and thought processes now than it did twelve years ago when this Alzheimer's nightmare began. As a seventy-five-year-old, I don't know how much time I have left—none of us does—and the only thing I'm sure of is that I have one less day in my life today than I did yesterday.

And then it hit me. I needed to say goodbye to the relationship Clair and I had enjoyed so much, cherished so much, in the pre-Alzheimer's chapters of our lives, because that part of us was gone, save for the memories that I still savoured. And that decision made sense. Yet I did *not* want to say—would *not* say—goodbye to Clair herself. She was *still* there, and by God, *I was too*. We were in a new and unpredictable, at times frustrating, chapter in our lives. She probably didn't know who I was anymore, yet like that man in the poem, I knew who she was. And out of all this turmoil I had developed a better sense of who *I* was.

I had learned that I am a person with or without a partner. I was a person *in utero* before I knew anyone, and today in my later years, after all that has happened to me, all that I have experienced, I am even more of a person. And in this mind-bending, mind-boggling, anguish-laden process I have been through, I have been given the chance to get more meaning and purpose out of my life than ever before. This chance means new opportunities for me, perhaps new work situations, maybe a geographical relocation, reconnecting with family and friends, and maybe in time a new romantic relationship in my life. I know Clair would want that for me.

Having said this, I acknowledge that I do not completely identify with the committed gentleman in the poem at the beginning of this chapter. Like me, he is in his later years—exactly how much later, I don't want to know. Yet I am not as patient as he. He is content, even grateful to be with his wife. I am grateful when I am with Clair, yet more conflicted than he is. I want a relationship with my wife, and at the same time I want a relationship that includes mutuality with sexuality—a relationship with both warmth and heat. I want understanding and empathy from someone, with someone.

August 12, 2014. My heart is missing Clair this evening as it feels the swoop and flow of time and all the distances she and I have covered, all the experiences we have shared separately and together. And I feel the physical, the temporal and the emotional distance from her.

Three weeks ago, I moved. I am still in the same building where Clair found an apartment for us about twelve years ago to complement our dream home at Halfmoon Bay—a dream now gone with her AD—but I now live six floors higher. It is a bachelor apartment, so compact that our queen-sized bed is just two feet away from me as I type these words. But this is *my* place. Not *our* place. I have taken another step (up and) away from Clair. In downsizing our things with the help of good friends, I realized that I was also beginning to downsize the relationship and the warm, loving partnership that we had shared for more than fifteen years before she became symptomatic.

Tonight I am alone as I look out onto the waters of Burrard Inlet. I am sad yet appreciative of this change in my emotional being, tasting if not savouring a sense of closure in my life. I have taken another step—though this time a fairly large step—in letting Clair go. If I have been resisting losing her to her AD, tonight I am yielding to the poignant nostalgia and the reality of the loss, to the cleaner, sharper edges and boundaries of no longer being with her ever again. Knowing this and accepting it.

And yet . . . even as I pride myself on having let her go, I look at my bed in my newfound bachelor's suite and I see that one half—traditionally Clair's side—is strewn with books—*New Yorkers*, journals and newspapers. I think I have said goodbye, but the bed—our bed—continues to remind me of her. I learned from Betsy that grief often or usually waxes and wanes but eventually diminishes to a bearable level. And special loves, such as I've experienced with Betsy and Clair, may never end.

Perhaps not unrelated to my feelings tonight is the fact that for the last few months I have been spending time with a new friend. As we edge cautiously if warmly around shared and overlapping possibilities between us, I am reminded that readiness is rarely a black-and-white phenomenon but almost always is felt and experienced within shades of grey, whether or not we are consciously aware of these feelings. I think I am more ready for a new partnership than I was about a year ago when I was dumped by the anxious mental health worker. But I know that some parts of me are more ready for a new relationship than others.

August 21, 2014. Clair has just finished eating lunch when I visit. I want to snuggle with her so badly, even though she has been confined to a wheelchair for some four to five weeks now. I ask her if she'd like to snuggle.

She says, "Sure."

I push her in her wheelchair to her room and, after setting off the bed alarm two or three times, manage to align the wheelchair next to her bed where I flop down. I reach out to hold her hand and she clasps mine warmly. We are quiet. Her eyelids are drooping, barely open, but she still seems to be awake.

As I lean over to kiss her, she says something softly. I ask her to repeat herself, something she rarely does anymore.

"It's over," she tells me again quietly.

I take a few minutes to absorb this news. Assuming she is talking about us, I try to think of something to reassure her that it is not over, that I am still there for her, yet realize this would be arguing with her.

"Well," I tell her at last, "thanks for the memories."

She smiles, almost but not quite laughing.

The best yardstick for measuring how good your choices have been when it comes to the decision to move on is probably how you feel today about what you decided to do or did about it yesterday. If you are sleeping well, not second-guessing yourself and your important decisions, and feeling and performing reasonably in your daylight hours while continuing to enjoy your life and your friends daily or weekly, you probably have done one or more things right. If, however, you are in doubt, phone your counsellor and ask for an early appointment. And if you are curious about physical symptoms, phone your GP today. Do not forget to be kind to yourself.

If you have decided to move on, you must make sure that your new partner or potential new partner understands the nature of your position—that is, that you are neither married nor single and that this state may last for some time, possibly many years. You must also be sure that she/he appreciates and understands the level at which you are in touch with your own ambivalence and how you are dealing with an array of emotional positions. Your strategies may include reaching out for help, sharing with trusted friends, enjoying spiritual support while privately praying or meditating, or finding a faith community that meets your spiritual, religious and social needs. At the same time, you will need to ask yourself some very important questions. Have you and your new partner talked in some depth about your level of readiness to participate in and contribute to a new and important relationship? Do your perceptions of your respective positions in life and love mostly agree or overlap? Are you able to share feelings of grief comfortably, including conflicts, mixed feelings and unhappiness in your life with this new person, while also feeling sincerely listened to?

Have you reached the point that you are comfortable in telling friends and family about your new relationship? A medium or high level of comfort in doing so suggests a healthy position. Hiding these new changes in your life from most or all of your circle of friends and family suggests that you are still stuck in some significant way, conflicted, ashamed or uncomfortable in your decision; it calls for rethinking. Immediately. If you are wrestling with persistently guilty feelings, you need to talk with a professional until you can fully understand and appreciate the source of these feelings and deal with them.

This is also the time to listen closely to your inner self. You will be getting an abundance of anxious advice from kindly, well-meaning friends and family, such as "Slow down!" or "What's taking you so long?" While it's okay to listen to them, it is very important to listen to yourself first. And be careful. The road through both grief and healing is cratered with anxious sidewalk superintendents, family members and friends who are convinced they know what is right for you and your grieving experience better than you do.

The point is, be prepared for an abundance of anxiety around you, much (though not all) of it from people who are not aware of their own anxious feelings about your loved one's dementia, how you are dealing with it and all its ramifications, how your relationship with your partner is faring and the likelihood of your becoming involved in a new important relationship. In my own experience, I have had a hard time distinguishing where the anxiety of my friends and concerned family members stops and mine begins. So I advise you to expect anxiety, hear it and listen to it. Just don't respond to it immediately. When in doubt, bounce it off a neutral party such as your best friend or your therapist.

Remember in this new life to keep your keepsakes near enough that you can reach for them when you want to be close to your loved one again—but not out on the table. In response to my deep grief over losing my late wife, Betsy, I wrote a memoir, *In Praise of Strong Women*. The experience and the memories associated with that project were somehow very comforting, but I also found sharing that book with my friends and family very satisfying. I no longer felt quite as alone or lonely. Savouring old photos of Betsy and me and our kids still reassures me, yet stops just short of gladdening me. Old love notes and poetry I wrote to Betsy—and to Clair—mean so much to me today.

To suggest that the arrival of any form of dementia into a marriage might be a gift would be concrete sophistry. My own journey with Clair through a dozen years of Alzheimer's disease has meant hand-to-hand combat in an inevitably losing battle. Yet in engaging this enemy head on, I have had many rewards. I know now I am a better person not only for having known Clair but also for having taken this journey with her, and in accepting the terms of battle laid down by this disease, I had an opportunity to become a warmer, kinder and wiser—although wearier—person. I learned that those of us who make up the army of spousal caregivers, while improving our partners' well-being and comfort level, can also model strength and valour and daring for others and help make the community of those wrestling with dementia a kinder and more enlightened place.

So what advice do I have for you who are just joining the ranks of spousal caregivers? First, get a diagnosis. It will bring clarity for both you and your partner because diagnosis is prognosis. This sharper focus may bring pain and dismay, but it also illuminates that murky area where the battle lines are drawn, and helps us make better use of the time allotted to us. Second, it is easy to fall into the punishing, altruistic trap that caregiving can become; by all means, give help, love and nurturance to your partner, but don't be deluded into thinking that you are the only one who can care for him or her. There is help out there in the form of medical and care services and support groups, but you must go and find them. They won't come looking for you.

Third, avoid the high rates of illness and early death within the caregiving community by taking care of yourself physically, emotionally and socially. You may unwittingly attempt to bury your own deep-seated grief, sadness, loneliness, frustration and even anger by working harder than ever, endangering your own health. Remember that whatever is good for your heart is good for your head.

Fourth, know that the road to positive, healthy caregiving is often lined with anxious friends and family members who are sometimes overly helpful, so your autonomy may be vulnerable. When you find yourself conflicted, get professional help.

Finally, remember that there is life for you after your partner's struggle with Alzheimer's. Your job is to find the balance for yourself, the equilibrium within the chaos that is—or was—your life, a balance that allows you to continue to grow, to nurture and love your partner while not limiting yourself to possibilities of newer, more dynamic, more bilateral forms of loving and partnering.

> **Saturday, September 6, 2014.** On this beautiful Indian summer afternoon I find my love asleep in her wheelchair, half-dressed with a shirt covering her nightgown, blankets strewn across her lap. Her mouth is agape and her head droops to the left.
>
> I start to waken her, think better of it and, pulling a chair over beside her, sit to enjoy the quiet closeness. I caress the nape of her neck tenderly then, concerned about waking her, desist. After a while she opens her eyes briefly and I move my head into her range of vision, even holding up a glass of cranberry juice for her. She looks through the glass and apparently through me, too. Her eyelids soften and she is asleep again—if she was ever awake— her head wilting farther to the left.
>
> I let myself out and walk out into the warm September afternoon sunshine.

Notes

Chapter One

1 K. Alagiakrishnan et al., "Montreal Cognitive Assessment Is Superior to Standardized Mini-Mental Status Exam in Detecting Mild Cognitive Impairment in the Middle-Aged and Elderly Patients with Type 2 Diabetes Mellitus," *BioMed Research International* 2013 (2013).

Chapter Two

1 Gabor Maté, *When the Body Says No* (Toronto: Knopf Canada, 2004), 158.

2 C.T. Loy et al., "Genetics of Dementia," *The Lancet* 383, no. 9919 (March 1, 2014).

3 D.A. Snowdon, "Healthy Aging and Dementia: Findings from the Nun Study," *Annals of Internal Medicine* 139, no. 5 (September 2, 2003).

4 "National Institute on Aging Renews Funding for UCI's 90+ Study" [news release October 17, 2013], *University of California Irvine News*, https://news.uci.edu/2013/10/17/national-institute-on-aging-renews-funding-for-ucis-90-study (accessed 2 October 2017).

5 J.C. Dooren, "The Best Foods for Thought, Literally," *Wall Street Journal*, February 14, 2012.

6 R. Krikorian et al., "Dietary Ketosis Enhances Memory in Mild Cognitive Impairment," *Neurobiology of Aging* 33, no. 2 (February 2012).

7 P. Fayerman, "Fighting Alzheimer's Starts in the Kitchen," *Vancouver Sun,* February 21, 2012.

8 "Can Coconut Oil Treat Alzheimer's?" *Berkeley Wellness,* June 1, 2012.

9 E.B. Ansell et al., "Cumulative Adversity and Smaller Gray Matter Volume in Medial Prefrontal, Anterior Cingulate, and Insula Regions," *Biological Psychiatry* 72, no. 1 (July 1, 2012).

10 M. Jameson, "Fear Dementia? Your Diet, Weight More Important Than Genes, Experts Say," *Orlando Sentinel*, January 24, 2012.

11 Ibid.

12 S. Alladi et al., "Bilingualism Delays Age at Onset of Dementia, Independent of Education and Immigration Status," *Neurology* 81, no. 22 (November 26, 2013): 1938.

13 M.J. Pontecorvo and M.A. Mintun, "PET Amyloid Imaging as a Tool for Early Diagnosis and Identifying Patients at Risk for Progression to Alzheimer's Disease," *Alzheimer's Research and Therapy* 3, no. 11 (March 2011): 6–7.

14 R.J. Bateman et al., "Clinical and Biomarker Changes in Dominantly Inherited Alzheimer's Disease," *New England Journal of Medicine* 367, no. 9 (August 30, 2012): 795.

15 T. Valeo, "Searching for the Early Signs of Alzheimer's Disease," *Neurology Now* 8, no. 5 (October–November 2012).

16 M.E. Mapstone et al., "Plasma Phospholipids Identify Antecedent Memory Impairment in Older Adults," *Nature Medicine* 20, no. 4 (March 9, 2014).

17 T. Lu et al., "REST and Stress Resistance in Ageing and Alzheimer's Disease," *Nature* 507, no. 7493 (March 27, 2014): 448.

18 H. Devlin, "Scientists Find First Drug That Appears to Slow Alzheimer's Disease," *The Guardian*, July 22, 2015.

19 Andrea Gillies, *Keeper: A Book About Memory, Identity, Isolation, Wordsworth and Cake* (New York: Broadway Books, 2009), 126–27.

20 D.E. Bredesen, "Reversal of Cognitive Decline: A Novel Therapeutic Program," *Aging* 6 no. 9 (September 27, 2014).

Chapter Three

1 C. Wilson, "Alzheimer Cafes Put Focus on the Person," Saint John *Telegraph-Journal*, January 16, 2012.

2 G.D. Cohen, "Anxiety in Alzheimer's Disease: Confusion and Denial," *American Journal of Geriatric Psychiatry* 6, no. 1 (Winter 1998): 2.

Chapter Five

1 A. Sauer, "Five Reasons Why Music Boosts Brain Activity," *Alzheimers.net*, https://www.alzheimers.net/2014-07-21/why-music-boosts-brain-activity-in-dementia-patients (accessed October 2, 2017).

2 M. Churchill et al., "Using a Therapy Dog to Alleviate the Agitation and Desocialization of People with Alzheimer's Disease," *Journal of Psychosocial Nursing and Mental Health Services* 17, no. 4 (April 1999).

Chapter Six

1 "Valuing the Invaluable: The Economic Value of Family Caregiving," *AARP Public Policy Institute*, https://assets.aarp.org/rgcenter/il/ib82_caregiving.pdf (accessed October 2, 2017).

2 Ibid.

3 S.E. Black et al., "Canadian Alzheimer's Disease Caregiver Survey: Baby Boomer Caregivers and the Burden of Care," *International Journal of Geriatric Psychiatry* 25, no. 8 (August 2010).

4 R.A. Beeson, "Loneliness and Depression in Spousal Caregivers of Those with Alzheimer's Disease Versus Non-Caregiving Spouses," *Archives of Psychiatric Nursing* 17, no. 3 (June 2003): 135.

5 S. Sanders et al., "The Experience of High Levels of Grief in Caregivers of Persons with Alzheimer's Disease and Related Dementia," *Death Studies* 32, no. 6 (July 4, 2008): 495.

6 J. Perry, "Wives Giving Care to Husbands with Alzheimer's Disease: A Process of Interpretive Caring," *Research in Nursing and Health* 25, no. 4 (August 2002): 307.

Chapter Seven

1 E.L. Ballard and C. Poer. *Sexuality and the Alzheimer's Patient* (Durham, NC: The Duke Family Support Program, Duke University Medical Center, 1993).

2 D.G. Harwood et al., "Prevalence and Correlates of Capgras Syndrome in Alzheimer's Disease," *International Journal of Geriatric Psychiatry* 14, no. 6 (June 1999).

3 R. O'Boyle, "Intimacy, Marriage and Alzheimer's Disease," *ElderCare Online* http://www.ec-online.net/Knowledge/Articles/intimacy.html (accessed October 2, 2017).

4 L. Todres and K. Galvin, "Caring for a Partner with Alzheimer's Disease: Intimacy, Loss and the Life That Is Possible," *International Journal of Qualitative Studies on Health and Well-Being* 1, no. 1 (2006): 50.

5 *Quality Dementia Care #6: Understanding Dementia Care and Sexuality in Residential Facilities*, Alzheimer's Australia, https://www.dementia.org.au/sites/default/files/20101001_Nat_QDC_6DemSexuality.pdf (accessed October 2, 2017).

6 J. Biscupic, "A New Page in O'Connor's Love Story," *USA Today*, November 13, 2007.

7 T. Parker-Pope, "Love, Divorce and Alzheimer's," *New York Times*, September 16, 2011.

8 A.M. Zeiss, H.D. Davies, M. Wood, and J.R. Tinklenberg, "The Incidence and Correlates of Erectile Problems in Patients with Alzheimer's Disease," *Archives of Sexual Behavior* 9, no. 4 (August 1990).

Bibliography

Books

Burdick, Lydia. *The Sunshine on My Face: A Read-Aloud Book for Memory-Challenged Adults.* Baltimore: Health Professions Press, 2004.

Denholm, Diana B. *The Caregiving Wife's Handbook: Caring for Your Seriously Ill Husband, Caring for Yourself.* Alameda, CA: Hunter House, 2012.

Doraiswamy, P. Murali and Lisa P. Gwyther with Tina Adler. *The Alzheimer's Action Plan: What You Need to Know—and What You Can Do—About Memory Problems, from Prevention to Early Intervention and Care.* New York: St. Martin's Griffin, 2008.

Gillies, Andrea. *Keeper: A Book About Memory, Identity, Isolation, Wordsworth and Cake.* New York: Broadway Books, 2009.

Kirkpatrick, David. *In Praise of Strong Women.* Vancouver: Granville Island Press, 2009.

Kling, Rabbi Simcha. *Reading IV from Yizkor—Memorial Service. Siddur Sim Shalom.* New York: The Rabbinical Assembly, 2005.

MacMillan, Angela, ed. *A Little, Aloud: An Anthology of Prose and Poetry for Reading Aloud to Someone You Care For.* London: Chatto & Windus, 2010.

Maté, Gabor. *When the Body Says No: The Cost of Hidden Stress.* Toronto: Knopf Canada, 2004.

Munro, Alice. *Hateship, Friendship, Courtship, Loveship, Marriage.* Toronto: McClelland & Stewart, 2001.

Peterson, Barry. *Jan's Story: Love Lost to the Long Goodbye of Alzheimer's.* Burlington, IA: Behler Publications, 2010.

Articles and Other Resources

Alagiakrishnan, K., N. Zhao, L. Mereu, et al. "Montreal Cognitive Assessment Is Superior to Standardized Mini-Mental Status Exam in Detecting Mild Cognitive Impairment in the Middle-Aged and Elderly Patients with Type 2 Diabetes Mellitus." *BioMed Research International* 2013 (2013): 1–5. https://doi.org/10.1155/2013/186106.

Alladi, S., T.H. Bak, V. Duggirala, et al. "Bilingualism Delays Age at Onset of Dementia, Independent of Education and Immigration Status." *Neurology* 81, no. 22 (November 26, 2013): 1938–44. https://doi.org/10.1212/01.wnl.0000436620.33155.a4.

Alzheimer's Disease: The Importance of Early Diagnosis [downloadable PDF]. Alzheimer Society of Canada. http://www.alzheimer.ca/~/media/Files/national/Core-lit-brochures/Importance_early_diagnosis_e.pdf (accessed October 2, 2017).

Ambiguous Loss and Grief: A Resource for Individuals and Families. Alzheimer Society of Canada.

Ansell, E.B., K. Rando, K. Tuit, et al. "Cumulative Adversity and Smaller Gray Matter Volume in Medial Prefrontal, Anterior Cingulate, and Insula Regions." *Biological Psychiatry* 72, no. 1 (July 1, 2012): 57–64. https://doi.org/10.1016/j.biopsych.2011.11.022.

Ballard, E.L., and C. Poer. *Sexuality and the Alzheimer's Patient*. Durham, NC: The Duke Family Support Program, Duke University Medical Center, 1993.

Bateman, R.J., C. Xiong, T.L.S. Benzinger, et al. "Clinical and Biomarker Changes in Dominantly Inherited Alzheimer's Disease." *New England Journal of Medicine* 367, no. 9 (August 30, 2012): 795–804. https://doi.org/10.1056/NEJMoa1202753.

Beeson, R.A. "Loneliness and Depression in Spousal Caregivers of Those with Alzheimer's Disease Versus Non-Caregiving Spouses." *Archives of Psychiatric Nursing* 17, no. 3 (June 2003): 135–43. https://doi.org/10.1016/S0883-9417(03)00057-8.

Belonogoff, L. "Talking about Intimacy, Sexuality and Alzheimer's." *In Touch* [newsletter of the Alzheimer Society of B.C.], June 2008.

Biscupic, Joan. "A New Page in O'Connor's Love Story." *USA Today*, November 13, 2007.

Black, S.E., S. Gauthier, W. Dalziel, et al. "Canadian Alzheimer's Disease Caregiver Survey: Baby Boomer Caregivers and the Burden of Care." *International Journal of Geriatric Psychiatry* 25, no. 8 (August 2010): 807–13. https://doi.org/10.1002/gps.2421.

Bredesen, D.E. "Reversal of Cognitive Decline: A Novel Therapeutic Program." *Aging* 6, no. 9 (September 27, 2014): 707–17. https://doi.org/10.18632/aging.100690.

"Can Coconut Oil Treat Alzheimer's?" *Berkeley Wellness*, June 1, 2012.

Churchill, M., J. Safaoui, B.W. McCabe, et al. "Using a Therapy Dog to Alleviate the Agitation and Desocialization of People with Alzheimer's Disease." *Journal of Psychosocial Nursing and Mental Health Services* 17, no. 4 (April 1999): 16–22.

Cohen, G.D. "Anxiety in Alzheimer's Disease: Confusion and Denial." *American Journal of Geriatric Psychiatry* 6, no. 1 (Winter 1998): 1–5.

Devlin, H. "Scientists Find First Drug That Appears to Slow Alzheimer's Disease." *The Guardian*, July 22, 2015.

Dooren, J.C. "The Best Foods for Thought, Literally." *Wall Street Journal*, February 14, 2012, D1.

Fayerman, P. "Fighting Alzheimer's Starts in the Kitchen." *Vancouver Sun* (February 21, 2012): A1.

Harwood, D.G., W.W. Barker, R.L. Ownby, et al. "Prevalence and Correlates of Capgras Syndrome in Alzheimer's Disease." *International Journal of Geriatric Psychiatry* 14, no. 6 (June 1999): 415–20. https://doi.org/10.1002/(SICI)1099-1166(199906)14:6<415::AID-GPS929>3.0.CO;2-3.

Jameson, M. "Fear Dementia? Your Diet, Weight More Important Than Genes, Experts Say." *Orlando Sentinel*, January 24, 2012.

Kirkpatrick, D. "Make Hay While the Sun Shines." *Canadian Medical Association Journal* 179, no. 8 (October 7, 2008): 803–4. https://doi.org/10.1503/cmaj.080681.

Krikorian, R., M.D. Shidler, K. Dangelo, et al. "Dietary Ketosis Enhances Memory in Mild Cognitive Impairment." *Neurobiology of Aging* 33, no. 2 (February 2012): 19–27. https://doi.org/10.1016/j.neurobiolaging.2010.10.006.

"Lilly Announces Top-Line Results of Solanezumab Phase 3 Clinical Trial" [news release November 23, 2016]. *Cision PR Newswire*. https://www.prnewswire.com/news-releases/lilly-announces-top-line-results-of-solanezumab-phase-3-clinical-trial-300367976.html (accessed 2 October 2017).

Loy, C.T., P.R. Schofield, A.M. Turner, et al. "Genetics of Dementia." *Lancet* 383, no. 9919 (March 1, 2014): 828–40. https://doi.org/10.1016/S0140-6736(13)60630-3.

Lu, T., L. Aron, J. Zullo, et al. "REST and Stress Resistance in Ageing and Alzheimer's Disease." *Nature* 507, no. 7493 (March 27, 2014): 448–54. https://doi.org/10.1038/nature13163.

Mapstone, M.E., A.K. Cheema, M.S. Fiandaca, et al. "Plasma Phospholipids Identify Antecedent Memory Impairment in Older Adults." *Nature Medicine* 20, no. 4 (March 9, 2014): 415–8. https://doi.org/10.1038/nm.3466.

"National Institute on Aging Renews Funding for UCI's 90+ Study" [news release October 17, 2013]. *University of California Irvine News*. https://news.uci.edu/2013/10/17/national-institute-on-aging-renews-funding-for-ucis-90-study (accessed 2 October 2017).

O'Boyle, R. "Intimacy, Marriage and Alzheimer's Disease." *ElderCare Online*. http://www.ec-online.net/Knowledge/Articles/intimacy.html (accessed 2 October 2017).

Parker-Pope, T. "Love, Divorce and Alzheimer's." *New York Times*, September 16, 2011.

Perry, J. "Wives Giving Care to Husbands with Alzheimer's Disease: A Process of Interpretive Caring." *Research in Nursing & Health* 25, no. 4 (August 2002): 307–16. https://doi.org/10.1002/nur.10040.

Pontecorvo, M.J., *and* M.A. Mintun. "PET Amyloid Imaging as a Tool for Early Diagnosis and Identifying Patients at Risk for Progression to Alzheimer's Disease." *Alzheimer's Research & Therapy* 3, no. 11 (March 2011): 1–9. https://doi.org/10.1186/alzrt70.

Quality Dementia Care #6: Understanding Dementia Care and Sexuality in Residential Facilities [downloadable PDF]. Alzheimer's Australia. https://www.dementia.org.au/sites/default/files/20101001_Nat_QDC_6DemSexuality.pdf (accessed October 2, 2017).

Sanders, S., C.H. Ott, S.T. Kelber, et al. "The Experience of High Levels of Grief in Caregivers of Persons with Alzheimer's Disease and Related Dementia." *Death Studies* 32, no. 6 (July 4, 2008): 495–523. https://doi.org/10.1080/07481180802138845.

Sauer, A. "Five Reasons Why Music Boosts Brain Activity." *Alzheimers.net.* July 21, 2014.

Smith, M. "Re-Inventing a Life." *In Touch* [newsletter of the Alzheimer Society of B.C.], 2005.

Snowdon, D.A. "Healthy Aging and Dementia: Findings from the Nun Study." *Annals of Internal Medicine* 139, no. 5 (September 2, 2003): 450–4. https://doi.org/10.7326/0003-4819-139-5_Part_2-200309021-00014.

Todres, I., *and* K. Galvin. "Caring for a Partner with Alzheimer's Disease: Intimacy, Loss and the Life That Is Possible." *International Journal of Qualitative Studies on Health and Well-being* 1, no. 1 (2006): 50–61. https://doi.org/10.1080/17482620500518085.

Valeo, T. "Searching for the Early Signs of Alzheimer's Disease." *Neurology Now* 8, no. 5 (October–November 2012): 34–5. https://doi.org/10.1097/01.NNN.0000421661.73296.d6.

"Valuing the Invaluable: The Economic Value of Family Caregiving" [downloadable PDF]. *AARP Public Policy Institute.* https://assets.aarp.org/rgcenter/il/ib82_caregiving.pdf (accessed 2 October 2017).

Wilson, C. "Alzheimer Cafes Put Focus on the Person." Saint John *Telegraph-Journal*, January 16, 2012, C1.

Zeiss, A.M., H.D. Davies, M. Wood, et al. "The Incidence and Correlates of Erectile Problems in Patients with Alzheimer's Disease." *Archives of Sexual Behavior* 19, no. 4 (August 1990): 325–31. https://doi.org/10.1007/BF01541927.

About the Author

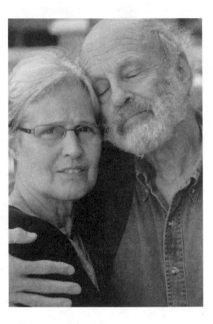

David Cowan Kirkpatrick, MA, MD, worked for forty years as a psychologist, psychiatrist and psychotherapist. He believes he works best when he acts as his patient's research assistant: "Better to help the patient sharpen the question than to provide or offer easy answers."

Raised in Yellow Springs, Ohio, the town that confused uniqueness with importance, he honed these interests and his particular philosophy since 1945. His perspectives were first shared in his IPPY award–winning book, *In Praise of Strong Women: A Psychiatrist's Memoir.* His love of women continues in the pages of his newly published second book, *Neither Married nor Single: When Your Partner Has Alzheimer's or Other Dementia.* In this book he invites his reader into the journey his wife and he shared through her long march through and battle with Alzheimer's disease, from both a personal and a professional perspective. It is one of the very, very few nonfiction books facing, exploring, addressing and dealing with the actual personal, emotional, physical, interpersonal, marital and sexual challenges, conflicts and other issues facing partners struggling with dementia in their relationships.